URBAN
CALISTHENICS

URBAN
CALISTHENICS

TEE MAJOR

ALPHA

CONTENTS

CALISTHENICS ESSENTIALS 9
Why Calisthenics? 10
The Benefits of Calisthenics 12
The Kaizen Philosophy 14
7 Simple Rules of Nutrition 16
Tips for Successful Training 18
Recovery, Injury
Prevention, and Rest 20
Equipment 22

WHOLE-BODY WORKOUTS 25
Build the Foundation 26
Brick by Brick 27
Bullet-Proof Core 28
Invictus 29
CRÆFT 30
All-4-1 31
Redistribution 32
True Grit 33
Popcorn-Ready 34
Nerves of Steel 35

PUSHING MOVEMENTS 37
Push-Up 38
Push-Up with Alternating
Leg and Arm Raise 40
Russian Push-Up 42
Pike Push-Up 44
Clapping Push-Up 46
Superman Push-Up 48
One-Arm Push-Up 50
One-Hand Clapping Push-Up............52
One-Arm, One-Leg Push-Up.............. 54
Dip to L-Sit 56
Triple-Clap Push-Up 58
Crucifix Push-Up 60
Handstand Push-Up......................62

PULLING MOVEMENTS 65
Bodyweight Row 66
Chin-Up 68
Pull-Up 70
Weighted Pull-Up 72
Commando Pull-Up 74
In-and-Out Grip Pull-Up.................76
Uneven Grip Pull-Up 78
Archer Pull-Up 80
Clapping Pull-Up 82
Muscle-Up 84
L-Sit Rope Climb 86
One-Arm Pull-Up 88

CORE MOVEMENTS 91
Hanging Knee Raise 92
Oblique Starfish 94
Hanging Leg Raise 96
L-Sit 98
Ab-Crunch Shredder 100
Buzzsaw 102
Headstand Leg Raise 104
Dragon Flag 106
Tuck Lever 108
Front Lever 110
Tuck Human Flag 112
Human Flag 114

CARDIO MOVEMENTS 117
Half Burpee 118
Skater 120
180 Rocket Jump 122
Carioca Run 124
Jumping Lunge 126
Burpee 128
Hurricane Burpee 130
Sumo Squat Jump 132
Box Jump 134
Lateral Hurdle Jump 136
Broad Jump 138
Box-to-Broad Jump 140
Double Broad Jump 142

LEG MOVEMENTS 145
Lunge 146
Side Lunge 148
Air Squat 150
Glute Bridge and March 152
Wall Sit 154
Elevated Single-Leg Glute Bridge.......156
Explosive Knee Jump 158
Hamstring Curl 160
Nordic Hamstring Curl 162
Shrimp Squat 164
Pistol Squat 166

WHOLE-BODY MOVEMENTS 169
Turkish Get-Up 170
Double-Leg Mountain Climber 174
Ninja Push-Up 176
Dragon Walk 178
Windshield Wiper 180
Flying Crow 182
Skin the Cat 184
Planche 186

INDEX 188

ABOUT THE AUTHOR 191

CREDITS 192

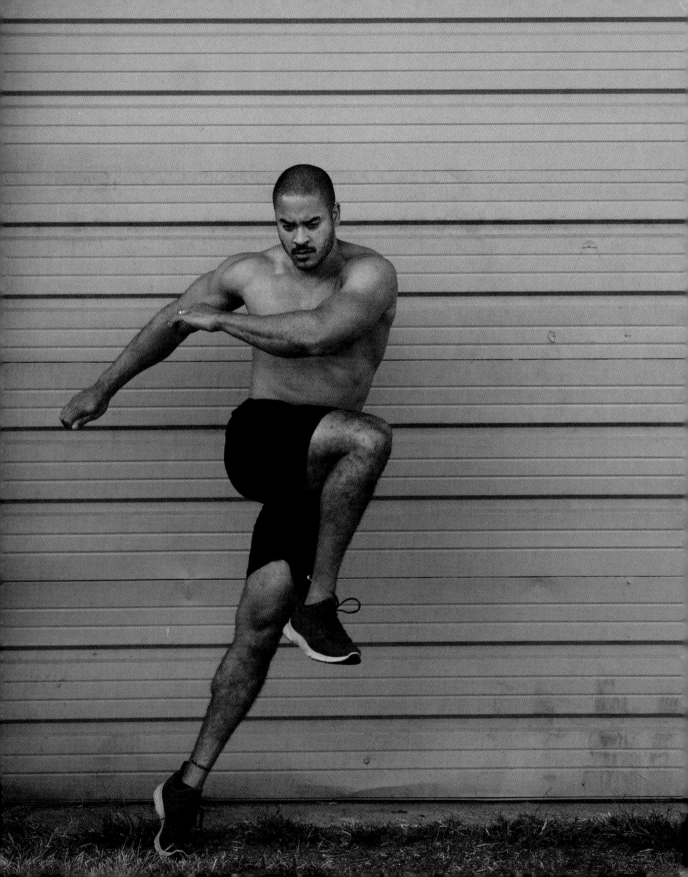

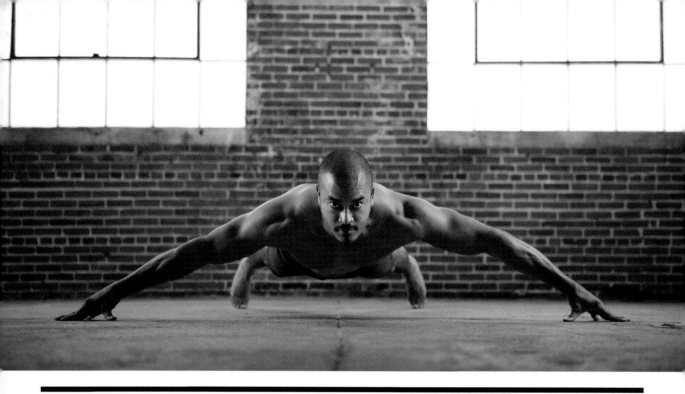

INTRODUCTION

Are you seeking a better way to get fit and strong? If you've picked up this book, you're already halfway there. Welcome to a better way to build a more complete self, both in body and in mind.

The U.S. military is made up of 1.2 million service members and an additional 800,000 volunteers, which means it's comprised of an incredibly diverse sampling of people from every corner of the country. There is, however, one thing nearly all of them have in common: they're very fit. Entry into these elite groups of protectors, where strength and fitness levels are reassessed every 6 to 12 months, requires personnel to spend weeks in boot camps where peak fitness is achieved, in part, through calisthenics.

I honed my calisthenics craft working with multiple branches of the U.S. military. Superior fitness is critical to a soldier's success. A soldier's mission might include a door-to-door patrol in enemy territory while carrying heavy gear and a rucksack,

or, as I know from working with troops in Kyrgyzstan, traversing steep mountain ranges to retrieve downed aircraft parts. For this reason, I decided to take my knowledge and apply it to training every branch of the military possible. My mission, simply put, was to maximize the athletic potential in all of my training partners so, no matter their mission, they were prepared.

My grandfather served in the military, and so did many of my uncles and cousins, and I've always been enamored with the discipline, structure, honor, and selflessness that every military member embodies, all of whom selflessly give themselves and their time to protect and serve those of us at home. However, underneath the "battle rattle," these men and women are just like you and me. On top of their jobs, they have duties to fulfill as mothers, fathers, brothers, and sisters. The lives of a military member and that of a civilian are both filled with everyday life struggles, but despite all of life's challenges, getting the job done no matter the circumstances, and reaching our full potential, is what the "warrior spirit" is about.

Over the years, my approach to training has evolved from using weight resistance and machines to mastering the art of calisthenics. Using the same methods outlined in this book, I was able to accomplish my "44 Best Bodyweight Exercises Ever!" video, which has garnered over 12 million views on YouTube. After I released "The 44" I embarked on a journey to learn as much about my mind and body as possible. I wanted to know what I was truly capable of, rather than settling for what I already knew I could accomplish. I viewed each training session as a learning experience—an opportunity for *Kaizen*, which is my adopted personal training philosophy. What I learned was that in order for us to reach our full physical potential, we need to approach our training with discipline, and we can never settle for mediocrity. We have a duty to realize our full human potential, and the more disciplined we are, the better the results will be. Plain and simple.

This book is written for *all* warriors, not just military, and it's designed to systematically elevate your fitness beyond what you've thought possible for yourself. The exercises and workouts in this book will help you develop strength and power, and reach your full potential, using only your mind and a few simple pieces of equipment. These methods have enabled countless men and women to extend their military careers and improve their physical test scores far beyond what they ever expected. They've also empowered men and women on the cusp of obesity and life threatening disease to improve their lives, and have given people of all backgrounds a higher quality of life, health, and performance. These methods can do the same for you.

Welcome to our journey.

Tee Major

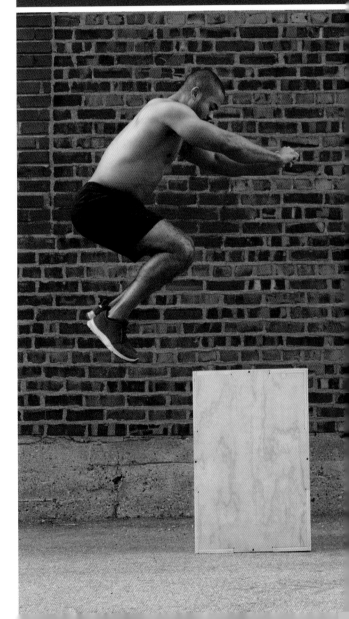

" We have a duty to realize our full human potential, and the more disciplined we are, the better the results will be. Plain and simple. **"**

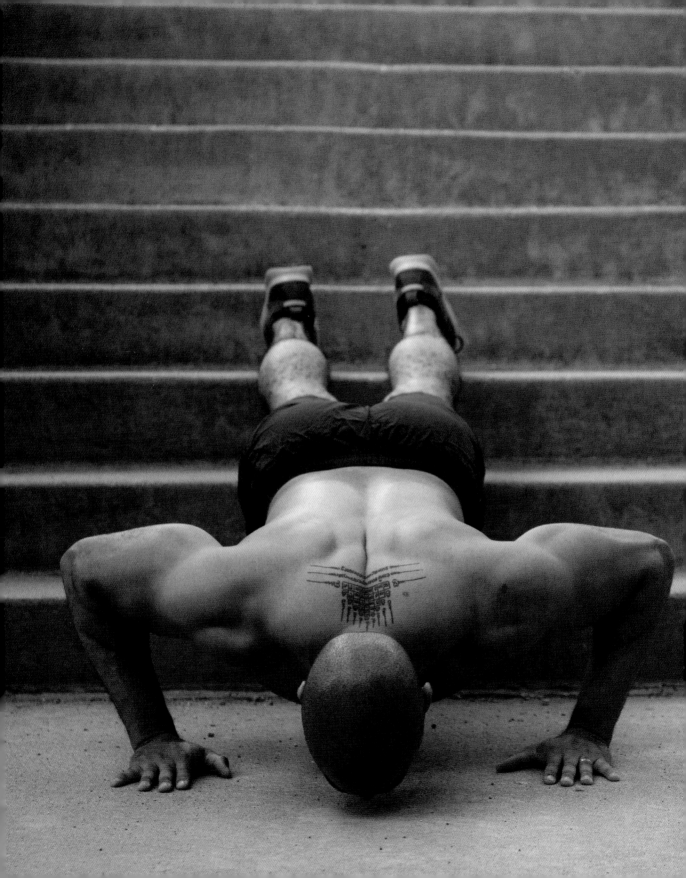

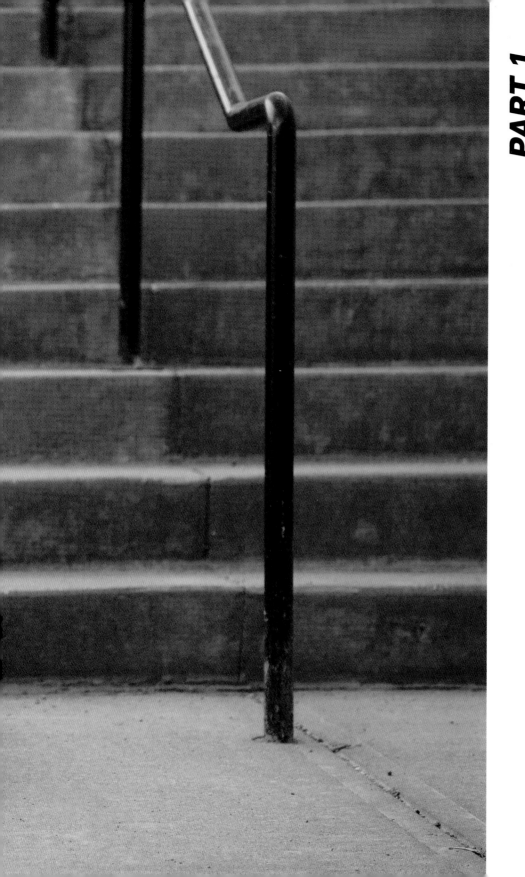

PART 1

CALISTHENICS ESSENTIALS

WHY CALISTHENICS?

When you hear the word "calisthenics," do you think of push-ups and pull-ups? I'm here to tell you that it's much more than that, and it's a better way to train.

A MODERN MOVEMENT...

Ironically, today's calisthenics movement was borne out of necessity. It all started in the streets and in urban environments, where people started using what was around them to get strong because they didn't have ready access to gyms and advanced equipment. Instead, bars in parks, flights of stairs, or ledges on buildings became the "equipment," and the urban environments where people lived became the "gyms." What people started to realize was they were getting incredibly strong, and also incredibly ripped, without a going to a gym or using expensive equipment. People soon realized they only needed simple environments and their own body weight to get as ripped and as strong as someone who was spending hours in a gym, and they were doing it in less time. What was once a necessity was now being embraced through a desire for simplicity and a deeper desire to free oneself from the confines of a gym. As the trend progressed, calisthenics gyms started popping up in parks across the U.S. and around the world, competitions sprouted and grew in number, and eventually calisthenic training became a movement. What was discovered was a new way to train that was simpler, more holistic, and faster than other, more commonly accepted methods of training.

...WITH ANCIENT ROOTS.

The roots of today's modern calisthenics movement took hold long ago. Before the days of gyms, humans built strong physiques through a more simplistic style of bodyweight training. Actions such as pushing, pulling, lifting, and other dynamic movements were natural components of everyday activities like farming or building, and these movements helped our ancestors build bodies that were strong, balanced, and functional. This ancient precursor to modern day training has been around since the Greeks coined the term ages ago. *Kallos,* which means "beauty," and *sthenos,* meaning "strength," are the roots of the modern term, and it's what defines the art form of using your own body weight to maximize human power and athletic ability. Centuries have passed, but the knowledge of the ancients has transcended time, and we can see and feel its influence in modern day systems of conditioning.

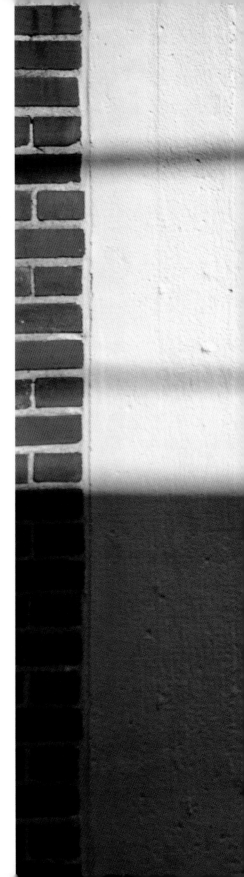

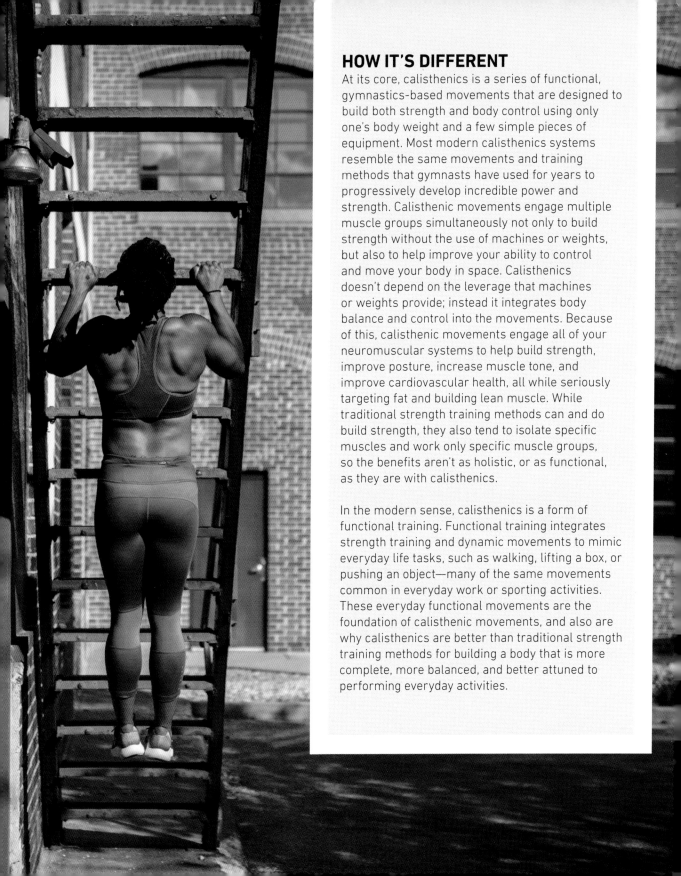

HOW IT'S DIFFERENT

At its core, calisthenics is a series of functional, gymnastics-based movements that are designed to build both strength and body control using only one's body weight and a few simple pieces of equipment. Most modern calisthenics systems resemble the same movements and training methods that gymnasts have used for years to progressively develop incredible power and strength. Calisthenic movements engage multiple muscle groups simultaneously not only to build strength without the use of machines or weights, but also to help improve your ability to control and move your body in space. Calisthenics doesn't depend on the leverage that machines or weights provide; instead it integrates body balance and control into the movements. Because of this, calisthenic movements engage all of your neuromuscular systems to help build strength, improve posture, increase muscle tone, and improve cardiovascular health, all while seriously targeting fat and building lean muscle. While traditional strength training methods can and do build strength, they also tend to isolate specific muscles and work only specific muscle groups, so the benefits aren't as holistic, or as functional, as they are with calisthenics.

In the modern sense, calisthenics is a form of functional training. Functional training integrates strength training and dynamic movements to mimic everyday life tasks, such as walking, lifting a box, or pushing an object—many of the same movements common in everyday work or sporting activities. These everyday functional movements are the foundation of calisthenic movements, and also are why calisthenics are better than traditional strength training methods for building a body that is more complete, more balanced, and better attuned to performing everyday activities.

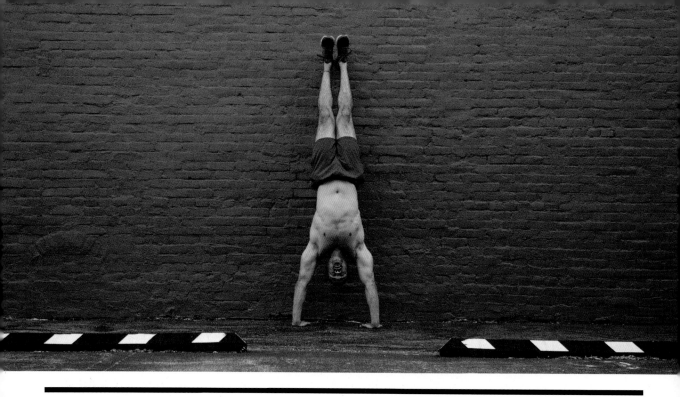

THE BENEFITS OF CALISTHENICS

The real beauty of calisthenics is that it builds an aesthetically pleasing body that also moves in a visually pleasing way. The calisthenics body is holistic, cohesive, and tenacious.

A STRONGER, MORE COMPLETE BODY

Calisthenic exercises are centered around dynamic functional movements, such as pushing and pulling, and these movements require you to utilize strength from your entire body, not just from one isolated muscle group. In addition, these movements also require stabilization and coordination to execute. This whole-body engagement results in a more complete development of your musculature, with the added benefits of increased strength, better coordination, and improved body control, all of which mean fewer injuries as you train. Another benefit is that soft tissue structures like tendons, ligaments, and fascia aren't as susceptible to the deconstructive, damaging, and unnatural movements of traditional resistance training; instead, they become stronger and more flexible. The strength and size of a body trained in the art of calisthenics are proportional because they're developed through authentic and natural movements, as opposed to movements that isolate specific muscles. Through calisthenics you'll experience improved coordination, speed, power, acceleration, strength, quickness, and agility. Bottom line, there is no mistaking a body built through calisthenics: it's strong, it's defined, and it's natural. And when certain movements are mastered, it's a magical thing to behold.

A HEALTHIER BRAIN

The mental and emotional benefits of exercise are well documented—exercise improves mood, fights depression, and helps regulate sleep patterns. But calisthenics has an added advantage over other forms of exercise: it works the brain as well as the body. Calisthenics exercises are the optimum demonstration of *psychomotor learning*, which is the complex interrelationship between cognitive function and physical movement. Driving a car, playing an instrument, and throwing a ball are all behavioral examples of psychomotor learning, where the brain and body have to work as one to learn and master an action. Because calisthenic movements engage multiple muscle groups while also requiring you to maintain balance and keep your body in control, the brain and body connection is enhanced.

Calisthenics also helps your brain and body work together to develop the fine motor skills necessary to perform complex tasks. This complex brain and body interplay, known as *proprioception*, is your brain's awareness of your body's position in space, as well as its recognition of the degree of effort required by the body to perform a specific task. This complex interplay helps fine tune our ability to perform everyday tasks. This enhanced connection may also help keep you lean. Once you begin training regularly in calisthenics, your subconscious mind will make the connection between functional movements and a leaner body composition to help regulate your appetite. People who take up calisthenics naturally drop fat and build muscle to develop more balanced, leaner physiques.

One thing is for certain, before you can perform any action effectively, you'd better be able to efficiently move your body through space. Calisthenics trains the body in a variety of ways to develop a blend of physical attributes that will help us move better, no matter the activity. While weights and machines can aid your balance, calisthenics requires that you also control your balance and engage mutiple muscle groups to do so. The result is a body that is trained more evenly than it would be through traditional strength-training methods.

> **❝All you need to get ripped and strong is your body, a few simple pieces of equipment, an environment where you can move, and the willpower to get it done.❞**

LESS EQUIPMENT, NO GYM

Because the majority of calisthenics movements are bodyweight-based, calisthenics requires very little equipment, and most movements don't require any equipment at all. A simple horizontal bar is all that's needed for most pulling exercises, while a stair step might be used for others. There are some basic pieces of equipment that will help make some moves even more effective, but the days of needing a gym with machines and weight plates are gone, as are the days of having to pay for an expensive gym membership, or for equipment that will end up collecting dust in your home. All you need to get ripped and strong is your body, a few simple pieces of equipment, an environment where you can move, and the willpower to get it done.

There's no arguing that calisthenics is gaining in popularity because of a trend towards minimalism. As we are afforded more and more luxury in these modern times, and accumulate more material goods that we don't always need, we can become more dependent on things, instead of ourselves. Instead of developing a sense of autonomy and independence, we might realize we are overwhelmingly restricted and isolated. However, by realizing we need less, we can realize we have more. The masters of martial arts, gymnastics, and calisthenics know this, and know that their bodies alone are their best tools for getting strong and ripped.

THE KAIZEN PHILOSOPHY

Kaizen is a Japanese philosophy for improvement, and it's what I've adopted and adapted as my personal philosophy and as a systematic way of conquering any challenge.

WHAT IS KAIZEN?

Roughly translated, *Kaizen* means "change for the better," or "improvement." The practical application of Kaizen emphasizes continuous improvement by making small changes, identifying and reducing waste (known as *muri*), and achieving greater goals by first setting and achieving smaller, incremental goals. When I started my calithenics journey, I thought about how I could achieve freedom from the confines of a gym. I wanted to strengthen every aspect of my body naturally, but also maximize the use of the space and time I had available. This required me to be flexible both in mind and body.

So, instead of looking for "bigger and better," I needed to look for more efficient and more meaningful. Through Kaizen I learned I can use less equipment, and utilize my body much more effectively and efficiently to build strength. And because I'm not tied to a gym or complicated equipment, I can train my body anywhere, and in less time. I'm a believer that in order to achieve your goals you need clarity, simplicity, and purpose, and because of Kaizen I've found I can train in less time, and with less effort. This is the Kaizen path to success—by needing less, we have more.

APPLYING KAIZEN TO CALISTHENICS

By applying Kaizen to calisthenics, you can take larger goals, like weight loss or strength gains, and break them down into smaller, more easily attainable goals. And by spotting and eliminating wasteful movements, or muri, you can make small, systematic improvements to help you reach those goals more quickly. If you begin by improving your form, you can perform movements more efficiently. And if you can perform movements more efficiently, you can master them more quickly and reach your training goals faster.

Kaizen follows no particular dogma, but there are a few integral components that are necessary for implementing it. I've found that the best way to implement Kaizen into your training is to boil it down into three simple steps.

1. EDUCATE

Begin by indentifying obstacles on your path to success. What muri exists in your training habits? What thoughts poison your mindset and mood and make you want to quit when you face an obstacle? What actions are harming your body? What foods are you ingesting that have little or no nutrition? Are you maximizing the time you have available to train? By first identifying small inefficiencies and bad habits, you can create strategies for eliminating muri, and also identify incremental goals that will help you make progress more quickly.

Shaolin monks practice the "empty mind" technique of meditation as a tool for clearing and focusing the mind, and it can work for you, as well. Achieving the "empty mind" and clearing your thoughts of clutter can be accomplished by performing a simple five-minute meditation each day. By reducing the clutter in your mind, you'll be better able to focus only on the task that lies in front of you without getting caught up in, and overwhelmed by, greater tasks or goals. You'll find that when you focus only on the task in front of you you'll be better able to embrace the Kaizen way.

[1] **Set a timer.** The Kaizen way is to incrementally build up to a goal, so start with one minute and gradually increase your time to five minutes as you become more comfortable with the process.

[2] **Ground yourself.** Seek a quiet location that is free of distractions. Lie flat on your back, sit cross-legged on the ground, or sit in a chair with your shoes removed and your feet flat on the ground. If you choose to sit, try to keep your back straight but without tensing up. (If you need to, you can sit against a wall.) If you choose to lie on the floor, find a comfortable location where you can stretch out comfortably.

[3] **Relax.** Close your eyes, and relax your shoulders, neck, and jaw. Take note of any areas of tension in your body, and focus on relaxing those areas.

[4] **Breathe deeply.** Focus on taking slow, controlled breaths through your nose. Notice how your breathing feels in the moment, and just breathe deeply and naturally.

[5] **Calm your mind.** Your mind may wander once you bring your focus to your breath. If this happens, simply bring your attention back to your breath. No matter how many times this happens, return to the moment by focusing on inhaling and exhaling.

2. ELIMINATE

Once you've identified the muri, you need to eliminate it strategically and purposefully. Are you not gaining the upper-body strength you expected? Focus on always keeping your lats engaged during pulling exercises. Is your form breaking down during pushing exercises? Double check hand and foot positioning to ensure they're correct. Focus exclusively on eliminating small, wasteful steps before moving on to the next movement. By making these small changes, you'll be better able to perform the movements that follow.

3. EVALUATE

This final step is about being in tune with your body and mindfully recognizing the changes that have occurred. How does the removal of the muri make you feel? Are you making the progress you feel you should be making? Are you gratified when you master a movement? Take the time to evaluate and document the changes, and acknowlege how the changes make you feel. It will help you reach your goals faster and help you enjoy the journey even more. Every small change is an improvement, and every improvement is an accomplishment.

7 SIMPLE RULES OF NUTRITION

A comprehensive calisthenics program is more than just dynamic movements, it also requires a sensible, disciplined approach to managing what you eat and when you eat it.

RULE #1
TREAT FOOD AS FUEL

The sooner you start treating food as fuel, the sooner you'll find yourself eating to build muscle and not eating to satisfy cravings. Eating a diet high in protein, complex carbohydrates, and good fats, and low in sugary carbs, sugar, and processed junk is a formula for success. Lean protein, such as lean meats and fish, helps heal and build muscle; complex carbohydrates, such as those found in whole grains, starchy vegetables, and beans, give you the fuel you need for powering through tough workouts; and healthy fats from sources such as olive oil and avocados, help heal cells and repair muscle tissue. Simple carbs from fruits help replenish spent glycogen stores.

RULE #2
DON'T STARVE YOURSELF

Starvation diets don't work. Anyone who has ever been on a starvation diet knows the pounds may come off quickly at first, but eventually you reach a point where you stop losing weight because your body enters starvation mode and begins storing fat. Fat storage is a natural survival mechanism, and it kicks in when we deprive our bodies of the minimum number of calories it needs to function properly. Since we burn even more calories when we exercise, we need to make sure we feed our bodies enough calories to function and fuel workouts, but not so many that our bodies convert those calories to fat. Eating too few calories can even cause your body to cannibalize its own lean muscle to get the nutrients it needs for survival.

RULE #3
HYDRATE

It's pretty simple. If you don't keep yourself properly hydrated, your body isn't going to perform at peak efficiency. By keeping yourself properly hydrated, your joints stay lubricated, your body is better able to regulate temperature and remove toxins, and it's better able to transport essential nutrients to organs and muscles. Dehydration can lead to cramping and dizziness, less efficient workouts, and serious health issues in extreme cases. Keep a water bottle full and handy at all times, and eat foods that are high in water content, such as cucumber, celery, melon, and grapefruit.

RULE #4
MANAGE YOUR METABOLISM

Your metabolism is the rate at which your body converts food to energy and burns fat, and it loves consistency. However, if you don't exercise regularly and eat three healthy meals and two to three snacks per day, the only consistent thing you will be able to count on will be a fluctuating insulin response because your body won't be able to figure out if you're starving or feasting. Eating at regular intervals helps keep your insulin levels consistent, and also means your body will get the full benefit of a metabolism that is burning fat at an efficient rate. Your metabolic efficiency is also directly related to the amount of activity you engage in each day. Following an exercise program in conjunction with a calorie-controlled diet will make your body even more efficient at losing fat and building muscle.

RULE #5
STAY OFF THE SCALE

As you begin your calisthenics journey, you'll find the fat disappears while the muscle grows. But how else can you measure your progress? While many people tend to step on the scale and obsess over a number, your Lean-Muscle-to-Body-Fat ratio (LBM) is a much more accurate barometer for measuring healthy body composition. LBM measures everything in your body besides the fat, including your bones, organs, muscle, and water. You can find calculators online to measure your LBM, but keep in mind that every person has a different ideal percentage of body fat, As a general rule, an average healthy body fat ratio is 18 to 22 percent for women and 15 to 17 percent for men. Women will start to look ripped when their LBM dips below 18%, while men will start to look ripped when their LBM dips below 13%.

RULE #6
EAT BREAKFAST

Breakfast truly is the most important meal of the day. Eating a nutritious breakfast gives us the fuel we need to get our bodies moving and helps fire our metabolism to help burn more calories and potentially help us lose weight faster. Studies have shown that eating breakfast helps regulate blood sugar levels, has a positive impact on fighting disease, and can even help improve cognitive function. Eating a full serving of protein first thing in the morning can prevent muscle catabolism, aid in muscle repair, and help curb hunger pangs long into the afternoon.

RULE #7
EAT WHOLE FOODS

This one is a no-brainer, but it's worth repeating: to build a healthy body, you need to eat a diet that includes whole grains, lean meats, and fresh fruit and vegetables. Processed foods, such as commercially baked goods, are poison and loaded with chemicals, preservatives, sugar, trans fats, and just about everything else that isn't good for you.

TIPS FOR SUCCESSFUL TRAINING

Getting the most out of your calisthenics training means you need to observe some best practices along the way. Patience, focus, and proper form are the keys. There are no short cuts.

FOLLOW THE PROGRESSION

Each chapter in this book is built upon the concept of starting with the first exercise in the chapter and moving on to the next only after you've mastered the one in front of you. Before you begin the progressions in each part, it will help to think of your body as a pyramid. You wouldn't build the top of the pyramid first, you would first build a strong foundation and then work your way up. Begin by visualizing what the pinnacle will look like, then start building the foundation, stone by stone, until you've reached a level where you can set that final stone at the top. Follow the Kaizen path as you begin your progressions, and perfect each and every step along the way as you master the most basic movements first, and don't move on to the next movement until you've mastered the one in front of you. To achieve the next level, you'll need to build an unbreakable and uncompromised foundation of strength in your shoulders, back, core, legs, and heart. Your training mantra should be to crawl first, walk second, and then run.

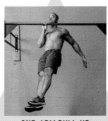

Building a pyramid
Mastering basic movements builds strength and stability for more advanced movements.

ONE-ARM PULL-UP

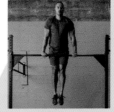

MUSCLE-UP

UNEVEN-GRIP PULL-UP

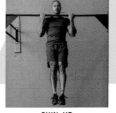

CHIN-UP

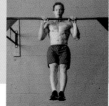

PULL-UP

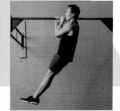

COMMANDO PULL-UP

PERFORM A DYNAMIC WARM-UP

Before you begin a workout, start by performing a dynamic warm-up that includes variations of squats, lunges, rotations, bridges, and core movements. Doing so helps prepare tendons, ligaments, joints, and the nervous system for safer, more successful training. The other benefit of performing a dynamic warm-up is that it helps break down the lactic acid that builds up in your muscles as you train, which is a common cause of soreness.

FOCUS ON BODY POSITIONING

No matter what type of training you've done previously, there isn't any substitute for perfecting the basics, and when it come to the basics of calisthenics, proper body positioning is *everything*. It can mean the difference between making progress and falling flat on your face or worse—injury. If you understand where every part of your body should be in the most basic movements, it will be much easier to accomplish the more advanced movements.

PACE YOURSELF AND VARY WORKOUTS

Hurriedly zipping through basic movements so you can master advanced movements is a surefire path to burnout or injury. If you're struggling to master a movement, try moving back to a previous movement and mastering that one again. You can also adjust your workload within training sessions, based upon how you're feeling and performing from day to day. At times, you may need to dial back a workout if you aren't feeling as strong and energized on any given day, even if it happens to be the same workout you performed on a previous day. It's important to push yourself, but also to know when to pull back. You should also vary your workouts to avoid injury. Training with variety and diversity of movement, and adding varying degrees of difficulties into your routines, will help keep you healthy and safe. Squeezing too many advanced exercises into one workout is a recipe for worn-out joints, damaged ligaments, and overly fatigued muscles. Just remember that what might be easy for one person might actually present a significant challenge for someone else, so listen to your body to determine what your maximum level of effort should be.

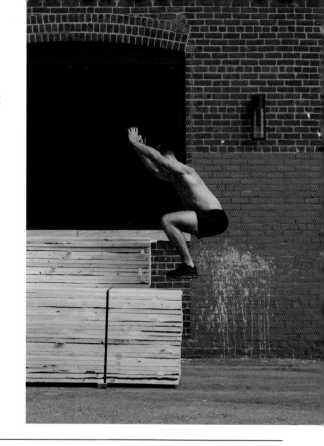

GRIND MODE *TRAINING SCALE*

The Grind Mode Training Scale is a simple system I've developed to help measure the perceived level of exertion required to execute an exercise or workout. Every workout and routine in this book is assigned a grind rating that reflects the perceived level of effort you'll need to exert in order to execute the movement or workout successfully. In the end, only you will know how much effort you'll need to exert in order to master a movement or finish a workout, but this scale will give you a general idea of what to expect as you move through the progressions.

GRIND MODE	DESCRIPTION
1-3 MILD GRIND	The level of exertion required will be relatively low. You may be able to talk as you perform the movements, and it may feel a bit more like play, but you will need to pay close to attention to form.
4-6 MODERATE GRIND	Things will become more difficult and it likely will take more time to master movements in this range. You will be noticeably more fatigued, and will also experience a higher degree of soreness.
7-8 STRONG GRIND	Things are getting serious. The movements in this range will be very difficult. It's likely you will feel significant fatigue and even exhaustion if you haven't built the proper foundation of strength.
9-10 MAX GRIND	Survival is questionable. The movements in this range are highly advanced and will take all your effort to execute. Your form may break down frequently, but if you've built the proper foundation, you will succeed.

RECOVERY, INJURY PREVENTION, AND REST

Every calisthenics program should follow a holistic approach that includes rest and recovery techniques for healing and rebuilding muscle tissue, and reducing the risk of injury.

RECOVERY TECHNIQUES

Muscle soreness can decrease performance and cause discomfort. Foam rolling, trigger pointing, and band stretching all can assist in breaking up knots, increasing blood flow, and restoring function to tight, sore muscles.

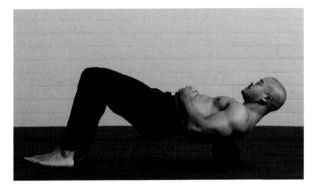

Foam rolling
Self-myofascial release, or foam rolling, can help alleviate soreness in muscles by applying pressure to specific areas to treat soft tissue restrictions. The sweeping motion of the roller combs over the muscle fibers to increase blood flow.

Trigger pointing
Trigger pointing muscles with a mobility ball can help remediate knots in tight muscles. By applying pressure to a particular area of the body, you can pinpoint sources of radiating pain and roll these points with a mobility ball.

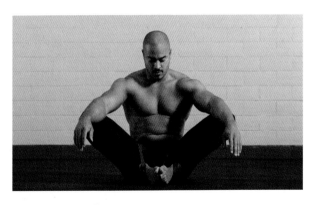

Band stretching
Using resistance bands for stretching is more effective than using static stretching methods alone. By using bands, you can perform dynamic stretches to stretch muscles through a greater range. Resistance bands can also be attached to bars or other objects for more dynamic stretches of legs, arms, and shoulders in order to help increase blood flow and restore range of motion in sore or tight muscles.

PREVENTING INJURIES

With frequent training, muscles can become knotted up like parachute cord. These knots can create tension and stretch a muscle at attachment points, which can lead to pain and injury. I've been fortunate to have had very few injuries over the span of my 20 years of training, and I attribute this to always diversifying my training and placing my body in unique and varying positions so I have a body that is balanced and strong. Bruce Lee aptly said, "Be like water." Simply put, work your body in a variety of positions to build a stronger, more complete foundation, and help avoid the unnecessary strain and stress that can lead to injury.

TIPS FOR **PREVENTING INJURIES**

- **Master the basics first** Once you've mastered the basic movements, chaining together muscle ups and front levers will come quite naturally and will become fun. However, trying to do too much and trying to do it too quickly is a recipe for injury. Build a solid foundation first.

- **Set realistic expectations** Whether you're just starting out or you've been training in calisthenics for a long time, you should let go of any ideas of perfection. We all want to become better athletes, but letting go of unrealistic expectations can help us define our own levels of success. Be present in the moment and embrace wherever you are today.

- **Pace yourself** Progressing to the next level before you're ready is setting yourself up for struggle and possible injury. Grind at a level that is fun, but still challenging enough to inspire you to come back to train another day. In the long run, you'll achieve your goals sooner and experience fewer setbacks.

TIPS FOR **BETTER SLEEP**

- **Be like Batman** Sleep in a dark room—as dark as you can get it. Unplug or cover electronics, and shut down computers.

- **Turn down the thermostat and bundle up** Your body needs to cool down in order to achieve restful sleep, and a cooler room will help you achieve that.

- **Stick to a set sleep schedule** Going to bed at the same time every night and waking up at the same time every morning helps keep you in tune with your body's circadian rhythms, which will lead to better rest.

- **Turn off the devices** Stop using electronics at least 30 minutes before bed. The blue light emitted from screens can interfere with the production of melatonin, which is the body's natural sleep hormone.

GETTING RESTFUL SLEEP

When you don't get enough sleep, your performance suffers, as does your body's ability to heal and build muscle. When you're fatigued, you have slower and weaker muscle contractions, so speed, power, and agility are negatively impacted. Additionally, your brain doesn't fire as fast and you have decreased memory retention, so reaction times and the ability to recall tasks is diminished. Plain and simple, you are a less athletic, slower thinking version of yourself when you don't get enough rest.

The optimal range for sleep is between 6 and 8 hours per night. As we sleep, our bodies cycle through lighter and deeper sleep cycles, and the deep sleep cycle is when our muscles relax, our heart rate slows, and our brain enters a dream state. It's also when we make the most "gains" because HGH (Human Growth Hormone) is released into the bloodstream to aid in muscle repair and development, so getting deep sleep is critical for proper muscle development.

EQUIPMENT

Most calisthenic movements only require your body weight to execute, but there are a few basic pieces of equipment that will help you train at peak efficiency.

FOAM ROLLERS

Foam rollers are just what they sound like—lightweight rollers made of high-density foam, and they're made for rolling targeted muscle areas for myofacial release. They come in a variety of sizes, and some are smooth, while others are textured for a more intensive release.

WHAT TO BUY Look for a durable, dent-resistant foam roller that is large enough to target every area of the body, but compact enough to travel.

KETTLEBELLS

Kettlebells are heavy, cast weights that resemble a ball with a handle. Unlike dumbbells, which are more conducive to pulling or pushing movements, kettlebells are ideal for swinging or ballistic (throwing) motions.

WHAT TO BUY Look for competition-grade kettlebells made of one piece of cast iron. Ideally you should have a variety of weights, but you can start with a lower weight if you're just starting out.

MOBILITY BALL

A mobility ball is a small hard rubber ball that is great for massaging trigger points and getting knots out of tight muscles. Using a mobility ball after particularly intense exercises can help speed up recovery and prevent tight muscles, which can lead to injury.

WHAT TO BUY Look for mobility balls that are made from natural rubber. (I'd advise you get a couple as these can come up missing quite often.)

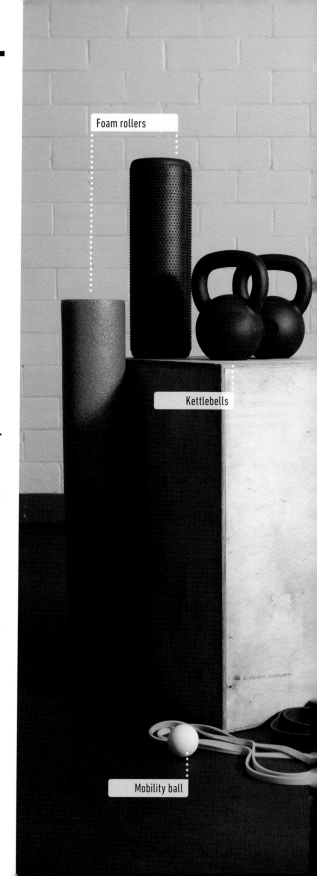

Foam rollers

Kettlebells

Mobility ball

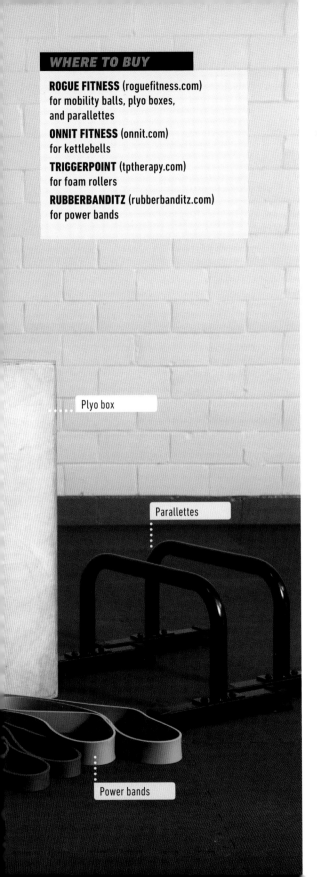

WHERE TO BUY

ROGUE FITNESS (roguefitness.com) for mobility balls, plyo boxes, and parallettes

ONNIT FITNESS (onnit.com) for kettlebells

TRIGGERPOINT (tptherapy.com) for foam rollers

RUBBERBANDITZ (rubberbanditz.com) for power bands

Plyo box

Parallettes

Power bands

PLYO BOX

A staple in many athletic training facilities, plyo boxes are sturdy, reinforced wooden boxes that offer a variety of heights for performing movements such as plyometric jumps, dips, or L-sits.

WHAT TO BUY If you're taller and well conditioned, start with a 20in (50cm) box. If you're shorter than average, deconditioned, or overweight, start with a shorter box, such as a 16in (40cm) box, and move up as your level of fitness improves. Look for a high-quality 3-in-1 box that can be flipped around to varying lengths and heights. Also, look for boxes with beveled edges (your shins will thank you if you happen to miss a jump).

PARALLETTES

Similar to the parallel bars you'd find in a gymnastics setting, parallettes are small, portable bars made of PVC plastic or steel, and are used for movements such as handstand push-ups or L-sits.

WHAT TO BUY At a minimum, parallettes should be slightly longer than shoulder width, stand high enough for performing L-sits, and be sturdy enough for handstand push-ups. Look for parallettes that measure at least 7 inches (17.5cm) from the top of the rail to the ground. The base should be long enough to prevent the parallettes from rocking or tipping over, and the length of the base should be proportional to the height.

POWER BANDS

Power bands are large, flat rubber bands that come in varying sizes and strengths. An important component of calisthenics is "muscle memory," which means that in order to master an exercise you have to practice it enough that your nervous system learns which muscles and energy systems it needs to activate in order to execute the movement. Power bands can assist muscle memory development by removing resistance and making it easier for your neuromuscular system to learn the proper body mechanics necessary to master a movement.

WHAT TO BUY Pick up a variety of resistance levels that will progress with you as your strength progresses. Look for strong, high-quality bands made through a layering process, not a casting process.

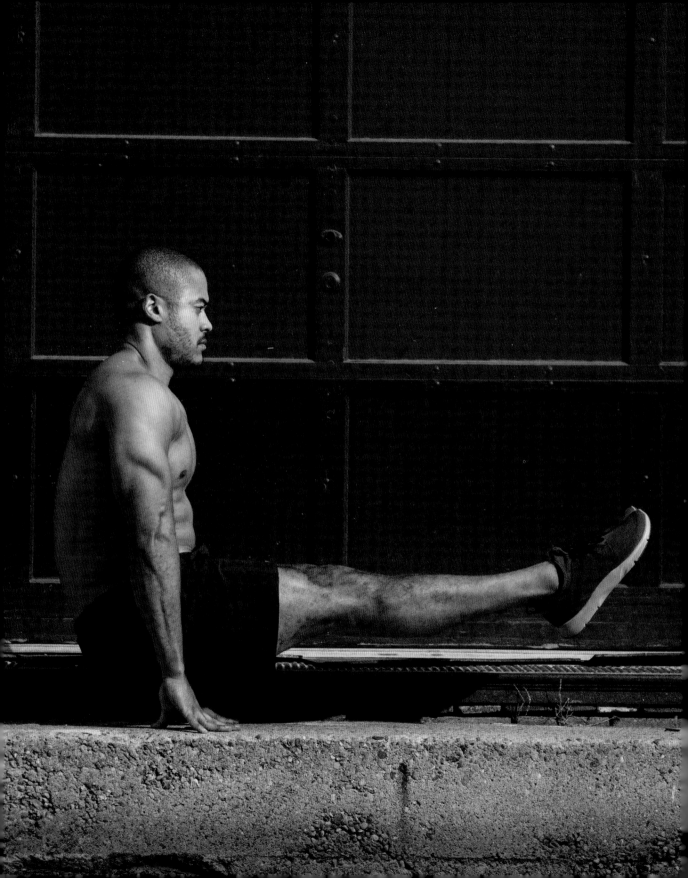

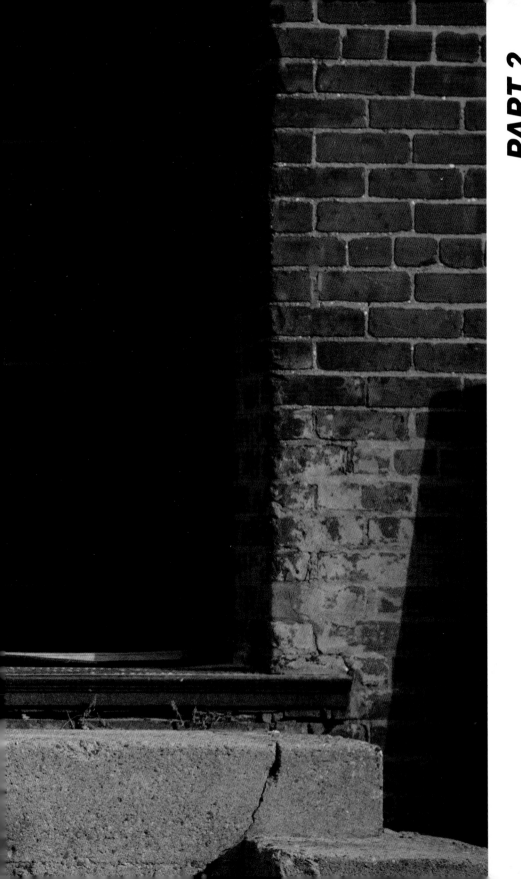

PART 2
WHOLE-BODY WORKOUTS

WORKOUT 1
BUILD THE FOUNDATION

There's no substitute for perfecting the basics. This workout will train each body part separately and build a foundation for the challenges ahead.

MOVEMENT	SETS	REPS/ TIME PER SET	REST BETWEEN SETS	PAGE
Push-Up	4	10 reps	30s	38
Bodyweight Row	4	10 reps	30s	66
Hanging Knee Raise	4	10 reps	30s	92
Lunge	4	10 reps per side	30s	146
Half Burpee	4	10 reps	30s	118

WARM-UP
mobility ball/foam rolling
(5 minutes)
dynamic warm-up (5 minutes)

COOL-DOWN
static stretching (5 minutes)

EQUIPMENT
horizontal bar

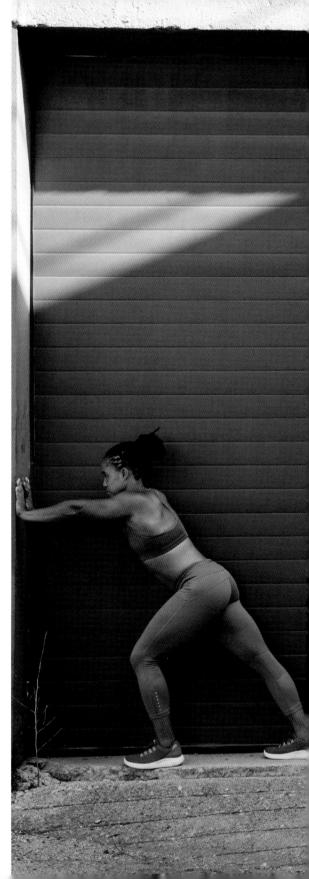

WORKOUT 2
BRICK BY BRICK

In this workout you will use variations of basic movements and some regression exercises to build a solid foundation of form, rep by rep, brick by brick.

MOVEMENT	SETS	REPS/ TIME PER SET	REST BETWEEN SETS	PAGE
Push-Up with Alternating Leg and Arm Raise	4	4 reps per side	45s	40
Pull-Up (band assisted)	4	8 reps	45s	70
Oblique Starfish	4	Hold for as long as possible	45s	94
Skater	4	8 reps per side	45s	120
Air Squat	4	8 reps	45s	150

WARM-UP
mobility ball/foam rolling
(5 minutes)
dynamic warm-up (5 minutes)

COOL-DOWN
static stretching (5 minutes)

EQUIPMENT
power bands

WORKOUT 3
BULLET-PROOF CORE

This core-shredding series includes a superset, which is simply a set that combines two exercises into one with no rest in between the movements.

MOVEMENT	SETS	REPS/ TIME PER SET	REST BETWEEN SETS	PAGE
Pike Push-Up	4	6 reps	1 min	44
Chin-Up	4	6 reps	1 min	68
(SUPERSET) Hanging Knee Raise Oblique Starfish	4	6 reps (3 reps per side) (Hold for as long as possible)	1 min	92 & 94
180 Rocket Jump	4	6 reps	1 min	122
Glute Bridge and March	4	6 reps	1 min	152

WARM-UP
mobility ball/foam rolling (5 minutes)
dynamic warm-up (5 minutes)

COOL-DOWN
static stretching (5 minutes)

EQUIPMENT
horizontal bar

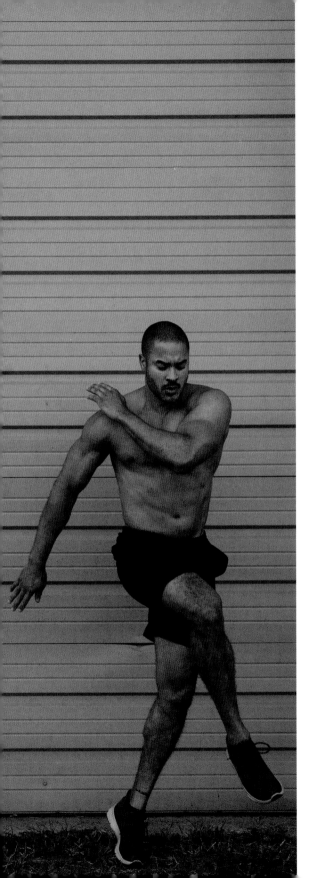

WORKOUT 4
INVICTUS

This series demands you prove you have earned your strength progression. Your grip, back, and core will all be tested, as will your coordination and balance.

MOVEMENT	SETS	REPS/ TIME PER SET	REST BETWEEN SET	PAGE
Russian Push-Up	4	10 reps	1 min	42
Pull-Up	4	10 reps	1 min	70
Hanging Leg Raise	4	10 reps	1 min	96
Glute Bridge and March	4	10 reps	1 min	152
Carioca Run (distance of 65 feet [20m] x 2=1 set)	4	10 reps	20s	124

WARM-UP
mobility ball/foam rolling
(5 minutes)
dynamic warm-up (5 minutes)

COOL-DOWN
static stretching (5 minutes)

EQUIPMENT
horizontal bar

WORKOUT 5
CRÆFT

Cræft is an old English word for the art and skill of strength. This workout utilizes the 3 classifications of strength: explosive, max, and endurance.

MOVEMENT	SETS	REPS/ TIME PER SET	REST BETWEEN SETS	PAGE
Clapping Push-Up	6	4 reps	1 min	82
Weighted Pull-Up	6	3 reps	1 min	72
L-Sit	6	Hold for as long as possible	45s	98
Wall Sit	6	1 minute	30s	154
Burpee	6	8 reps	30s	128

WARM-UP
mobility ball/foam rolling
(5 minutes)
dynamic warm-up (5 minutes)

COOL-DOWN
static stretching (5 minutes)

EQUIPMENT
horizontal bar

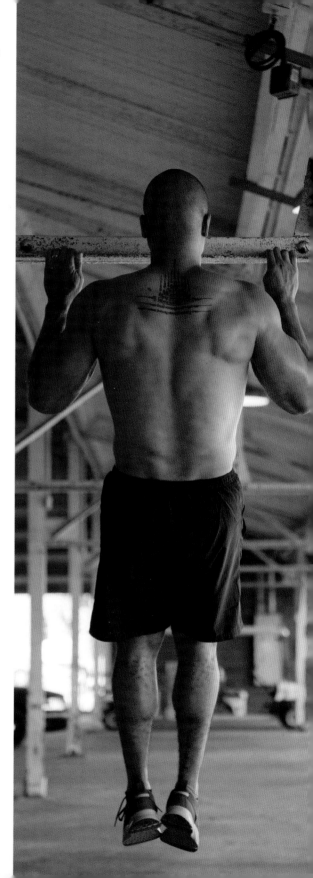

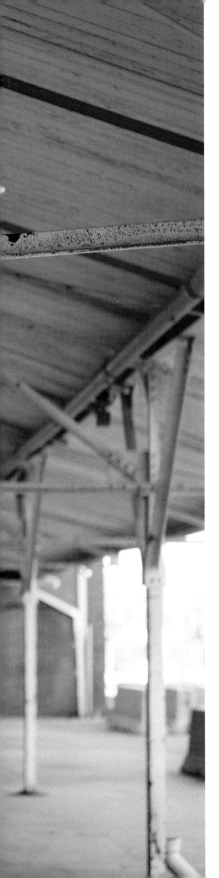

WORKOUT 6
ALL-4-1

Perform 4 reps for 1 goal: total body strength!
Group A movements are practiced for sets 1 and
2, and group B for sets 3 and 4.

	MOVEMENT	SETS	REPS/ TIME PER SET	REST BETWEEN SETS	PAGE
GROUP A (SETS 1 AND 2)	Clapping Push-Up	2	4 reps	1 min	46
	Weighted Pull-Up	2	4 reps	1 min	72
	L-Sit	2	Hold for as long as possible	1 min	98
	Wall Sit	2	1 minute	30s	154
	Burpee	2	4 reps	30s	128
	Turkish Get-Up	2	4 reps per side	1 min	170
GROUP B (SETS 3 AND 4)	Russian Push-Up	2	4 reps	1 min	42
	Pull-Up	2	4 reps	1 min	70
	Hanging Leg Raise	2	4 reps	1 min	96
	Glute Bridge and March	2	4 reps	1 min	152
	Carioca Run (distance of 65 feet [20m] x 2=1 set)	2	2 reps	20s	124
	Turkish Get-Up	2	4 reps per side	1 min	170

WARM-UP
mobility ball/foam rolling (5 minutes)
dynamic warm-up (5 minutes)

COOL-DOWN
static stretching (5 minutes)

EQUIPMENT
horizontal bar,
kettlebell,
dumbbell

WORKOUT 7
REDISTRIBUTION

This series creates a grinding workout by emphasizing movements that redistribute your weight between limbs to make the movements harder.

MOVEMENT	SETS	REPS/ DISTANCE PER SET	REST BETWEEN SETS	PAGE
One-Arm Push-Up	4	4 reps per arm	2 min	50
Uneven-Grip Pull-Up	4	5 reps	2 min	78
Buzzsaw	4	4 reps	1 min	102
Hamstring Curl	4	5 reps	1 min	160
Box Jump	4	8 reps	30s	134
Dragon Walk	4	10 meters	1 min	178

WARM-UP
mobility ball/foam rolling
(5 minutes)
dynamic warm-up (5 minutes)

COOL-DOWN
static stretching (5 minutes)

EQUIPMENT
horizontal bar,
plyo box, towel

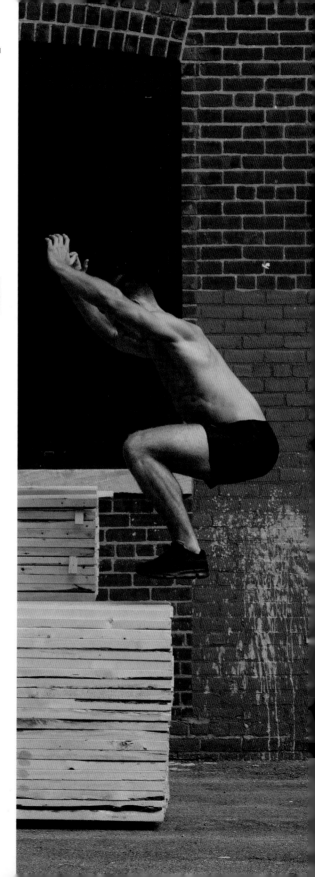

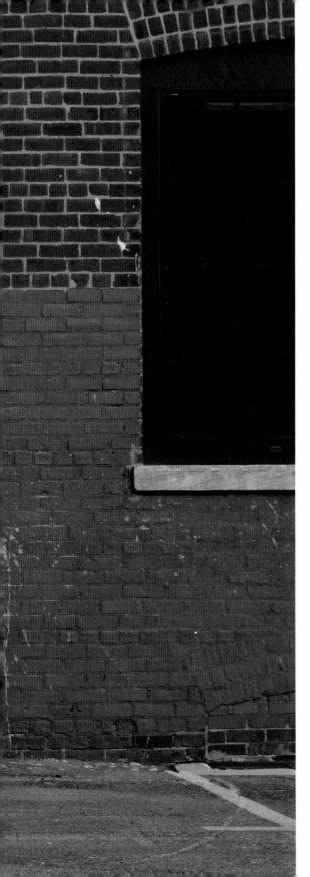

WORKOUT 8
TRUE GRIT

This workout features compound movements that are essential for building the strength necessary for the most advanced movements in this book.

MOVEMENT	SETS	REPS/ TIME PER SET	REST BETWEEN SETS	PAGE
Dip To L-Sit	5	5 reps	1 min	56
Muscle Up	5	5 reps	1 min	84
Headstand Leg Raise	5	5 reps	1 min	104
Nordic Hamstring Curl	5	5 reps	1 min	162
Broad Jump	5	5 reps	1 min	138
Flying Crow	5	Hold for as long as possible	1 min	182

WARM-UP
mobility ball/foam rolling
(5 minutes)
dynamic warm-up (5 minutes)

COOL-DOWN
static stretching (5 minutes)

EQUIPMENT
horizontal bar,
plyo boxes or
parallettes

WORKOUT 9
POPCORN-READY

I call this one popcorn-ready because people will want to stop and watch as you perform these serious calisthenics feats of strength.

MOVEMENT	SETS	REPS/ TIME PER SET	REST BETWEEN SETS	PAGE
One-Arm, One-Leg Push-Up	4	3 reps per side	2 min	54
Uneven-Grip Pull-Up	4	3 reps per side	2 min	78
Dragon Flag	4	4 reps	2 min	106
Shrimp Squat	4	5 reps per side	2 min	164
Box-to-Broad Jump	4	5 reps	2 min	140
Skin the Cat	4	3 reps	2 min	184

WARM-UP
mobility ball/foam rolling (5 minutes)
dynamic warm-up (5 minutes)

COOL-DOWN
static stretching (5 minutes)

EQUIPMENT
horizontal bar, plyo box, rings, towel

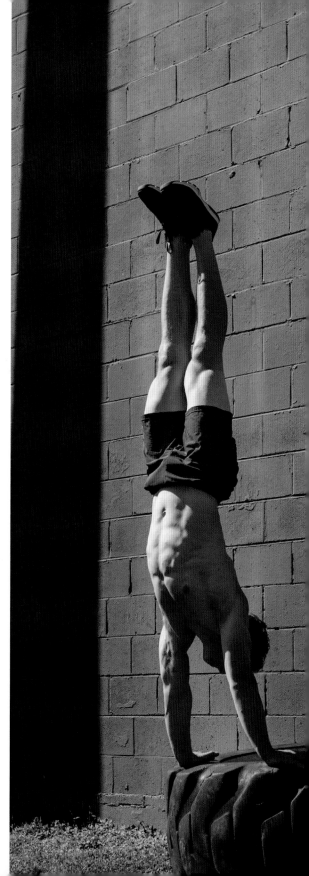

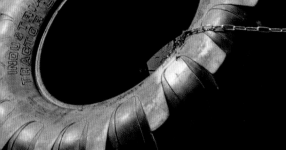

WORKOUT 10
NERVES OF STEEL

You really will need nerves of steel for this one. This series will test all your training up to this point, as well as your resolve for overcoming adversity.

MOVEMENT	SETS	REPS/ TIME PER SET	REST BETWEEN SETS	PAGE
Handstand Push-Up	3	3 reps	3 min	62
Uneven-Grip Pull-Up	3	3 reps per side	3 min	78
Tuck Human Flag	3	4 reps per side	3 min	106
Pistol Squat	3	5 reps per side	2 min	164
Double Broad Jump	3	5 reps	2 min	140
Planche	3	3 reps	3 min	184

WARM-UP
mobility ball/foam rolling (5 minutes)
dynamic warm-up (5 minutes)

COOL-DOWN
static stretching (5 minutes)

EQUIPMENT
horizontal bar, vertical bar, parallettes

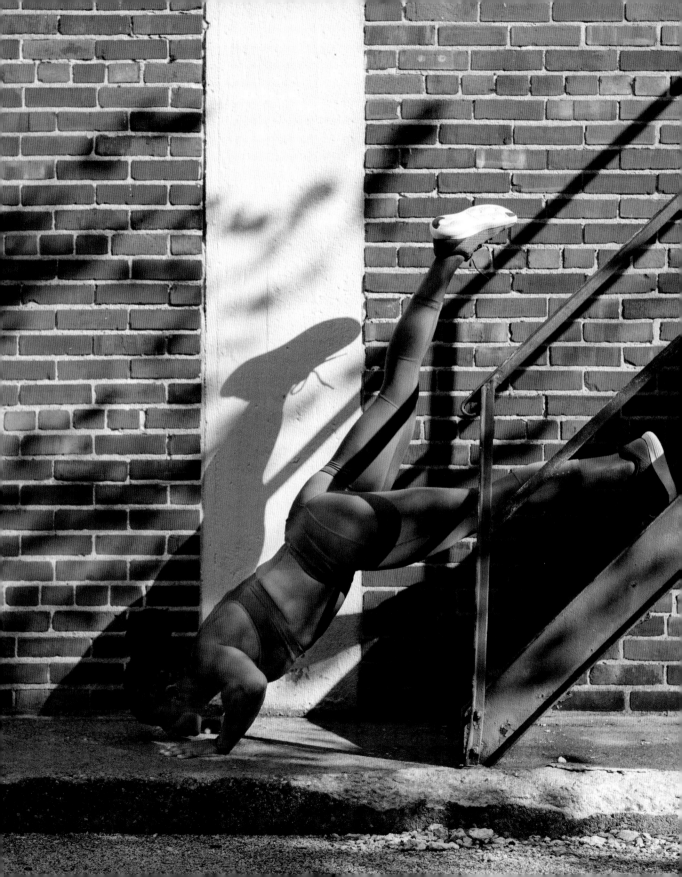

PART 3
PUSHING MOVEMENTS

PUSH-UP

The Push-Up is near and dear to my heart and is a foundational movement of calisthenics. And while the Push-Up doesn't look complicated, maintaining proper form is critical.

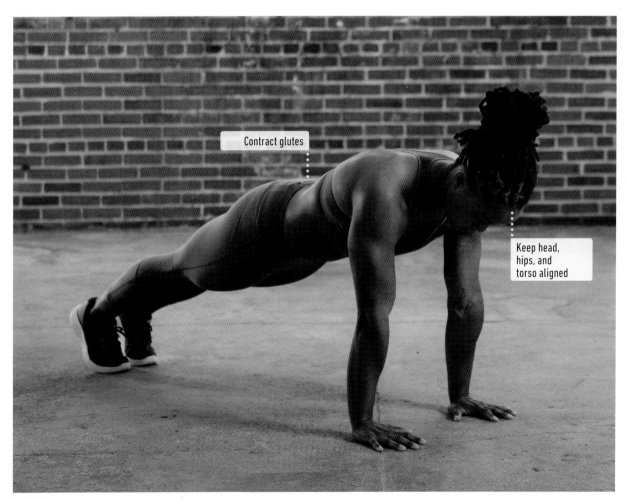

Contract glutes

Keep head, hips, and torso aligned

[1] Begin in a high plank position with your arms locked, your hands positioned slightly wider than shoulder width apart, and your fingers pointing forward. Push your shoulders down and away from your ears, and keep your abs and glutes tight.

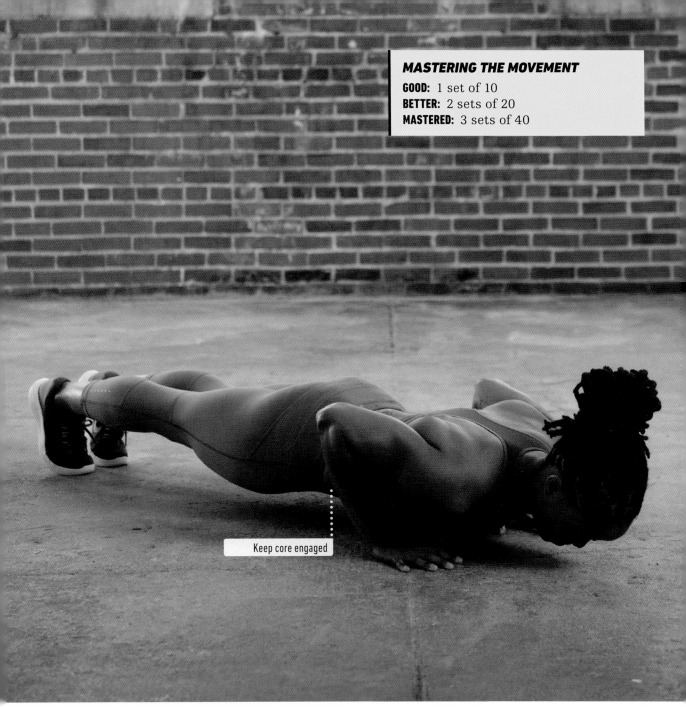

MASTERING THE MOVEMENT

GOOD: 1 set of 10
BETTER: 2 sets of 20
MASTERED: 3 sets of 40

Keep core engaged

[2] Drop into a low push-up position until your chest is just above the floor and your elbows are bent at 45-degree angles; then quickly push yourself back up into the starting position.

PUSH-UP WITH ALTERNATING LEG AND ARM RAISE

This variation is excellent practice for executing the One-Arm Push-Up. Good core strength is essential for keeping your body straight and lifting alternating limbs off the ground.

[1] Begin in a high plank position with your arms locked, your hands positioned slightly wider than shoulder width apart, and your fingers pointing forward. Push your shoulders down and away from your ears, and keep your abs and glutes tight.

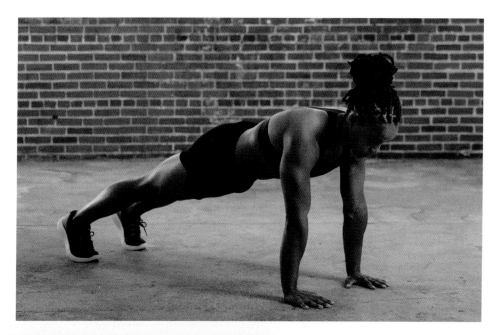

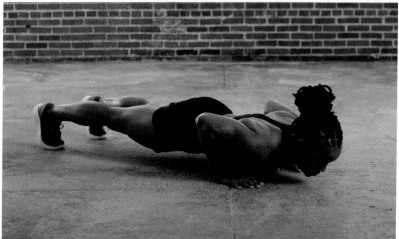

[2] Drop into a low push-up position until your chest is just above the ground and your elbows are bent at 45-degree angles.

[3] Quickly and explosively push yourself up while simultaneously lifting and extending your left arm and right leg off the ground.

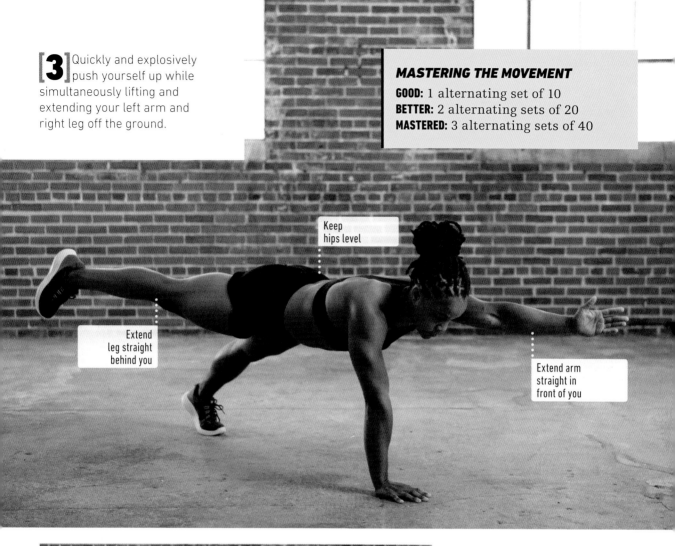

Keep hips level

Extend leg straight behind you

Extend arm straight in front of you

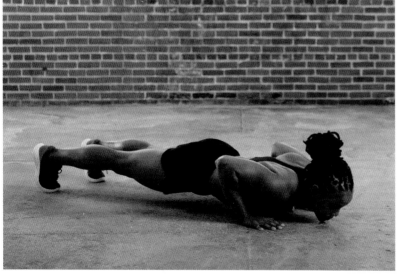

[4] Drop back into a low push-up position; then push yourself back up again while lifting and extending the opposite arm and leg off the ground.

RUSSIAN PUSH-UP

The Russian Push-Up is a fantastic movement for strengthening shoulders, biceps, and triceps in preparation for the more challenging push-up variations to come.

[1] Begin in a high plank position with your arms locked, your hands positioned slightly wider than shoulder-width apart, and your fingers pointing forward. Push your shoulders down and away from your ears, and keep your abs and glutes tight.

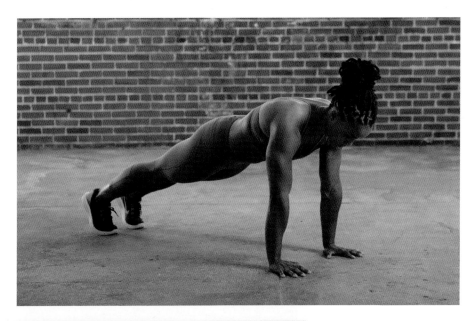

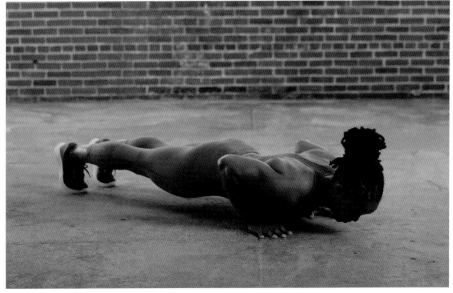

[2] Drop into a low push-up position until your chest is just above the floor and your elbows are bent at 45-degree angles.

[3] Rock your body backward by pushing through your palms and lowering your forearms to the ground.

MASTERING THE MOVEMENT

GOOD: 1 set of 10
BETTER: 2 sets of 20
MASTERED: 3 sets of 40

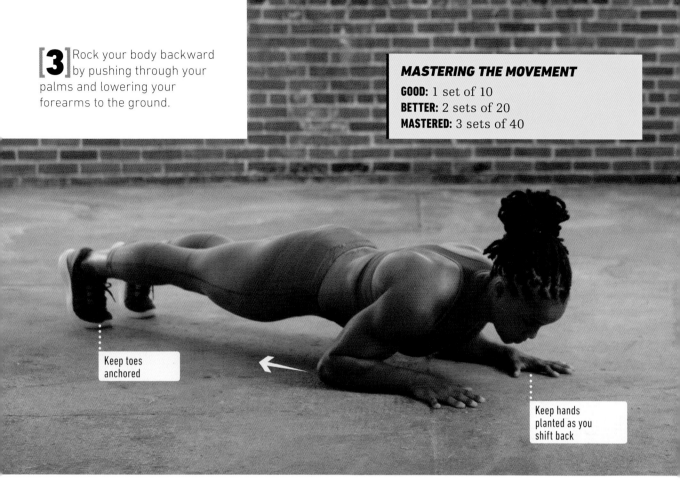

Keep toes anchored

Keep hands planted as you shift back

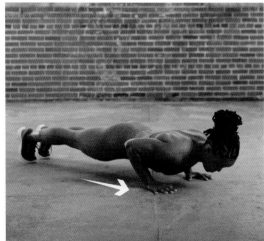

[4] Push through your palms and toes to rock your body forward and back into the low push-up position.

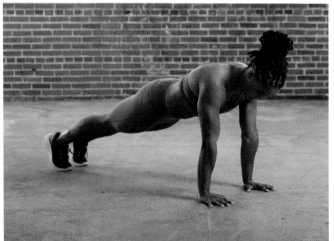

[5] Quickly push yourself back up into the starting position.

PIKE PUSH-UP

The Pike Push-Up will increase your shoulder strength and improve your core stability. The vertical-press positioning is excellent training for more complex calisthenics movements.

[**1**] Begin in a narrow-stance, high plank position with your elbows locked, your hands positioned slightly wider than shoulder-width apart, and your fingers pointing forward with your thumbs positioned directly below your ears. Push your shoulders down and away from your ears, and keep your abs and glutes tight.

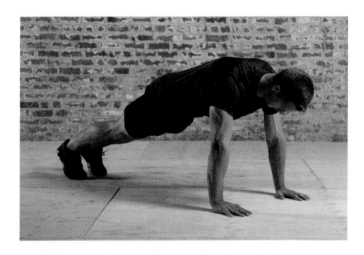

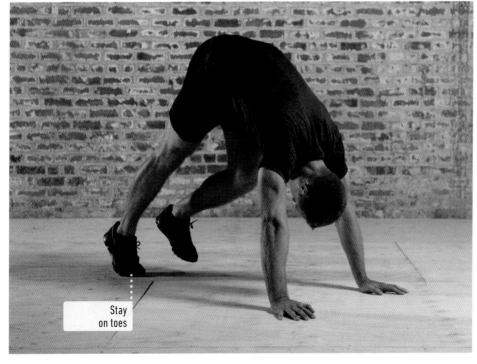

[**2**] Begin walking forward by taking small steps while simultaneously raising your hips vertically.

Stay on toes

[3] Continue walking forward as far as possible until your hips are over your feet, and your upper body and lower body are aligned in a pike position at a 90-degree angle.

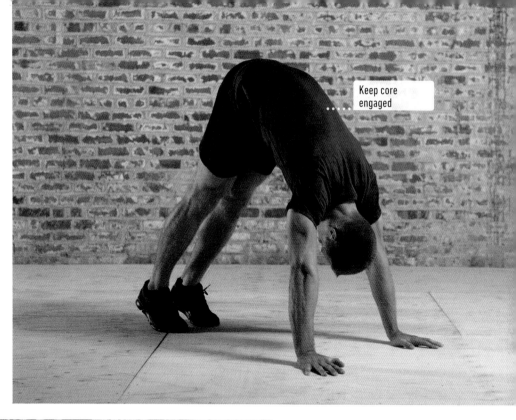

Keep core engaged

[4] Lower your body down into a push-up, and then push back up into the pike position.

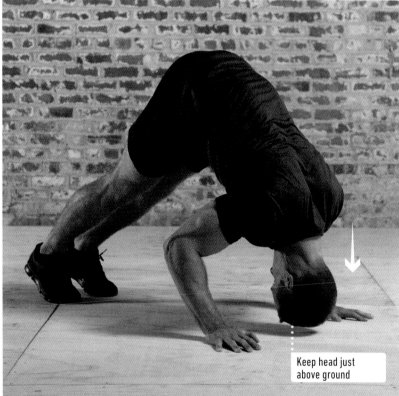

Keep head just above ground

MASTERING THE MOVEMENT

GOOD: 1 set of 10
BETTER: 2 sets of 20
MASTERED: 3 sets of 20

CLAPPING PUSH-UP

Nothing builds quick reflexes and dynamic pushing power like the Clapping Push-Up. This plyometric move will increase your ability to push heavy objects or throw a punch with great force.

[1] Begin in a high plank position with your hands positioned shoulder width apart and placed directly below your shoulders. Position your feet slightly closer than shoulder width apart.

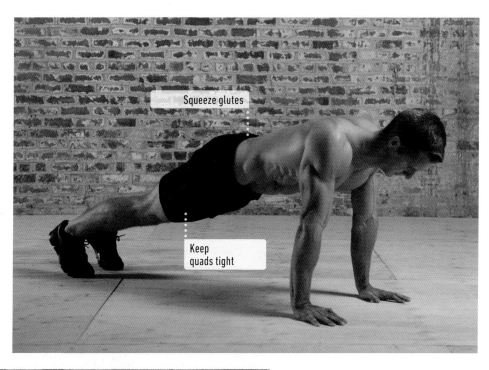

Squeeze glutes

Keep quads tight

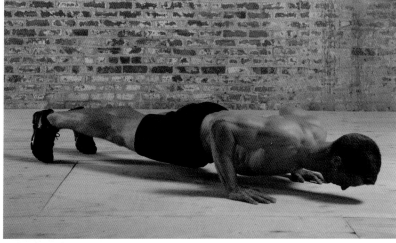

[2] Drop into a low push-up position, keeping your body just above the ground.

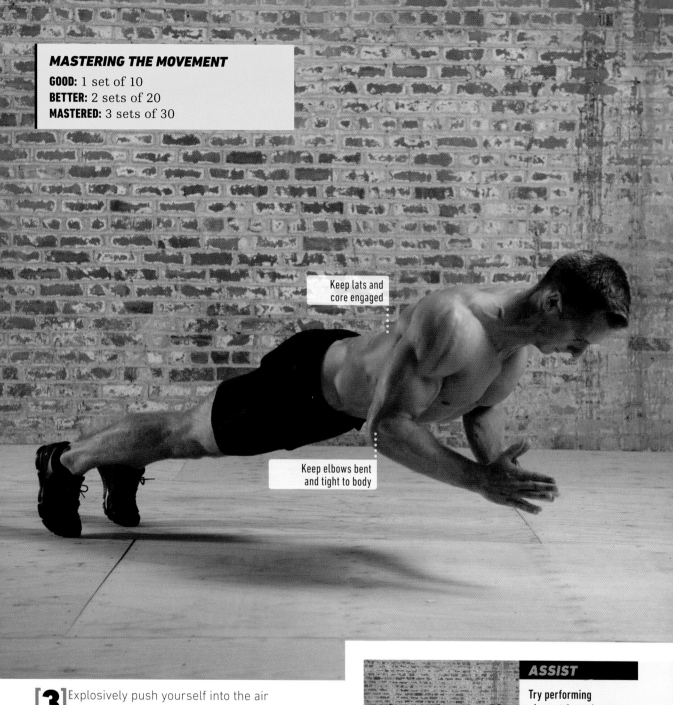

MASTERING THE MOVEMENT
GOOD: 1 set of 10
BETTER: 2 sets of 20
MASTERED: 3 sets of 30

Keep lats and core engaged

Keep elbows bent and tight to body

[3] Explosively push yourself into the air as high as possible, simultaneously performing a quick clap as you ascend, and then quickly return your hands to the ground as you descend back into a low push-up position.

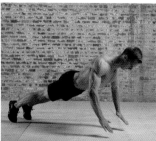

ASSIST

Try performing plyometric push-ups without a clap; then try clapping with your hands positioned on an elevated surface, such as stairs or a plyo box.

SUPERMAN PUSH-UP

This movement requires you to push your entire body weight into the air while lifting all of your limbs off the ground. Visualize yourself as Superman flying over Metropolis!

[1] Begin in a high plank position with your feet in a narrow stance, your arms locked, your hands positioned slightly wider than shoulder width apart, and your fingers pointing forward. Push your shoulders down and away from your ears, and keep your abs and glutes tight.

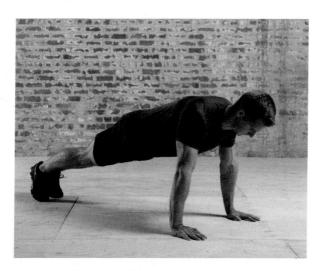

TIP
Perform on a mat or carpet before trying on a hard surface.

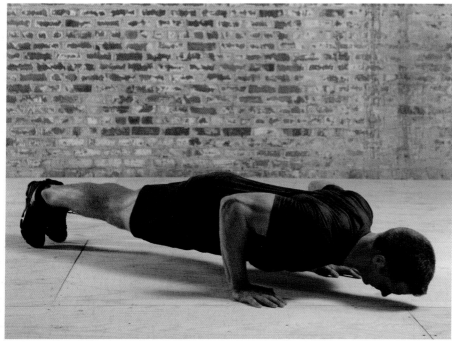

[2] Quickly lower yourself into a low push-up position, keeping your chest just off the ground.

MASTERING THE MOVEMENT

GOOD: 1 set of 3
BETTER: 2 sets of 4
MASTERED: 3 sets of 5

[3] Immediately explode skyward, raising your hands and feet up and away from your body as you ascend; then immediately bring your arms back down to execute a smooth landing on your toes and hands.

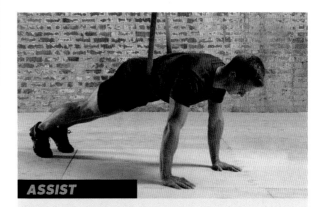

ASSIST

Try this first with a power band and bar assist. You can also start with a wider stance to minimize kipping at the hips.

ONE-ARM PUSH-UP

The One-Arm Push-Up is no common feat of strength and is fantastic for building raw power in your shoulders, chest, and triceps, in addition to stabilizing and strengthening your core.

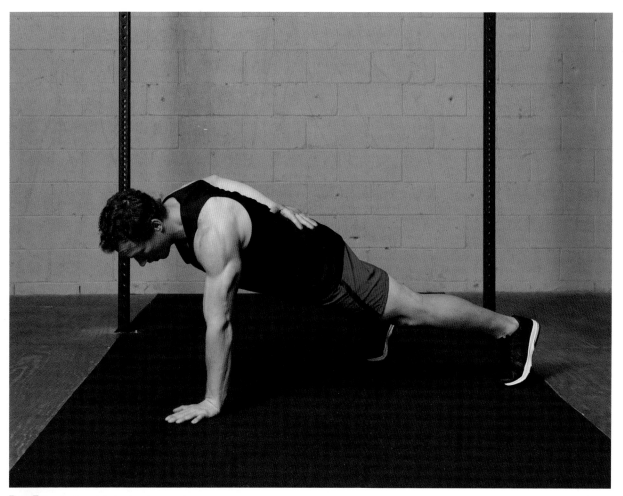

[1] Begin in a high plank position with one arm extended and locked, your hand placed flat on the ground and positioned just inside of your shoulder, and your fingers pointing forward. Place the opposite arm behind your back. Position your feet just slightly wider than shoulder width apart.

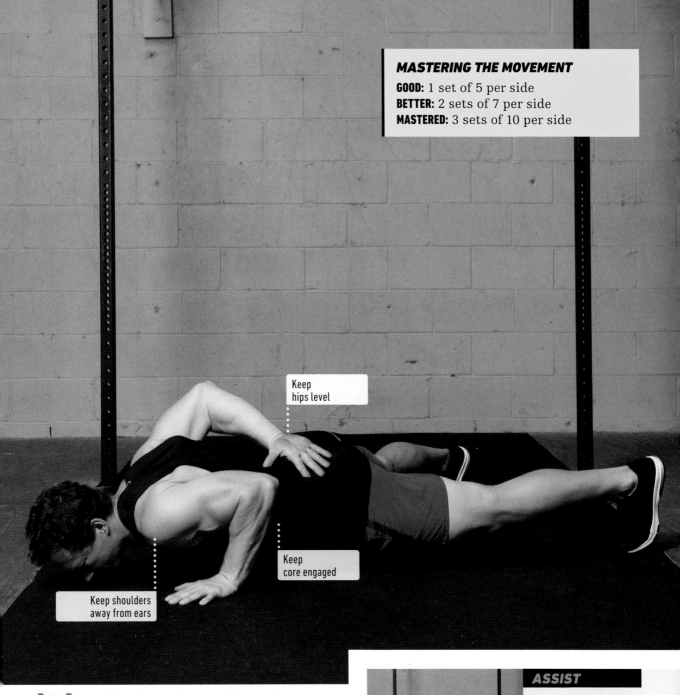

MASTERING THE MOVEMENT

GOOD: 1 set of 5 per side
BETTER: 2 sets of 7 per side
MASTERED: 3 sets of 10 per side

Keep
hips level

Keep
core engaged

Keep shoulders
away from ears

[2] Drop into a low push-up position until your chest is just above the ground and your elbow is bent at a 45-degree angle. "Corkscrew" your hand into the ground, and then immediately push through your hand to explode your body skyward and back into the high plank position.

ASSIST

Place your hand on a plyo box, a stack of weight plates, or a yoga brick before trying this one flat on the ground. Increasing the incline decreases the difficulty.

ONE-HAND CLAPPING PUSH-UP

A sure-fire way to make a push-up more challenging is to remove an arm from the equation and add a clap. When you've accomplished this one you've ventured into elite territory!

[1] Begin in a high plank position with one arm extended and locked, your hand placed flat on the ground and positioned just slightly inside of your shoulder, and your fingers pointing forward. Place the opposite arm behind your back and position your feet just slightly wider than shoulder width apart.

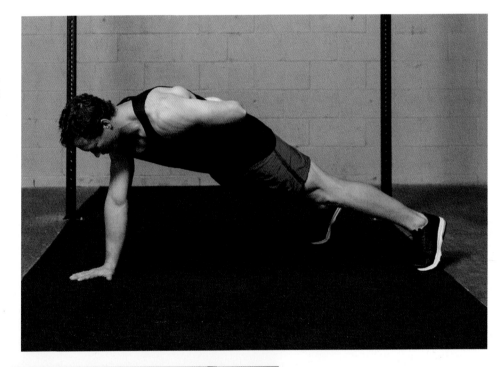

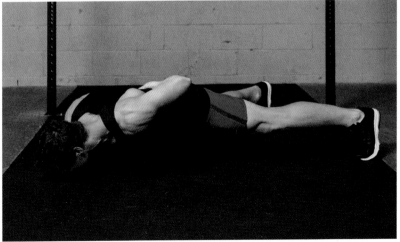

[2] Slowly lower your body into a low push-up position until your chest is just above the ground, and your elbow is bent at a 45-degree angle.

[3] "Corkscrew" your hand into the ground, and then immediately explode skyward while simultaneously performing a single clap as you ascend.

MASTERING THE MOVEMENT

GOOD: 1 set of 2 per side
BETTER: 2 sets of 3 per side
MASTERED: 3 sets of 5 per side

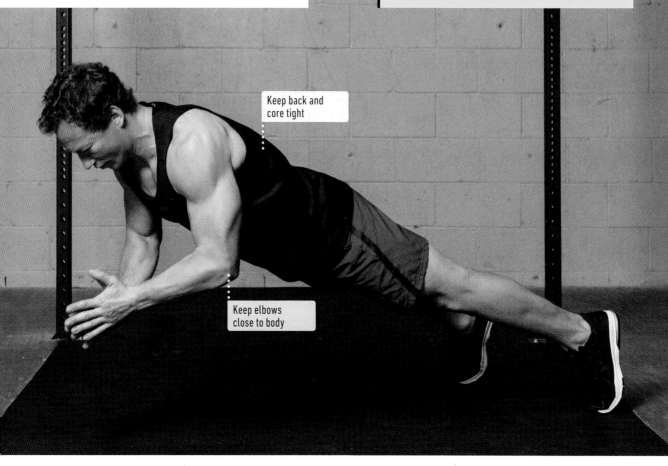

Keep back and core tight

Keep elbows close to body

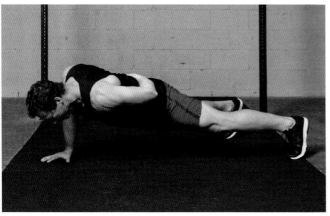

[4] Immediately place your non-pushing arm back behind you as you descend and land softly on your pushing hand.

ONE-ARM, ONE-LEG PUSH-UP

If you're ready for it, it's time to tackle this rarely seen, rarely executed push-up. This one really requires exceptional core strength, so make sure your abs are ready for the challenge!

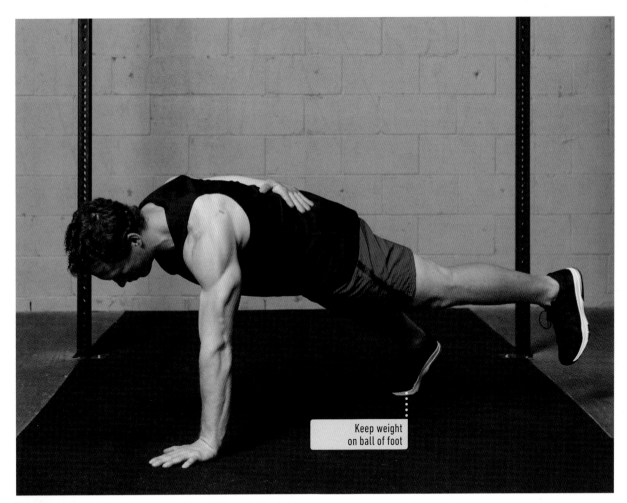

Keep weight on ball of foot

[1] Begin in a high plank position. Extend and lock your left arm with your hand placed flat on the ground and positioned just inside your shoulder, and your fingers pointing forward. Place your right arm behind your back. Position your feet in a wide stance, and lift and extend your left leg off the ground.

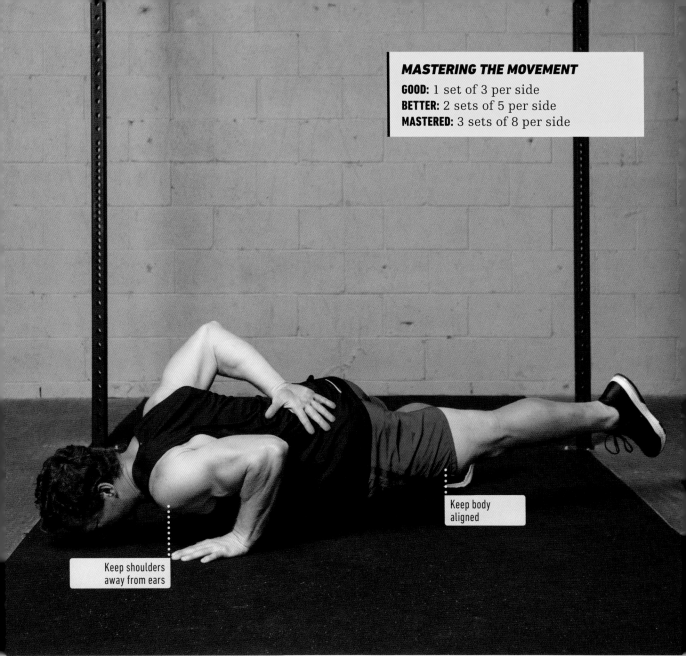

MASTERING THE MOVEMENT

GOOD: 1 set of 3 per side
BETTER: 2 sets of 5 per side
MASTERED: 3 sets of 8 per side

Keep body
aligned

Keep shoulders
away from ears

[2] Lower your body into a low push-up position until your chest is just above the ground and your elbow is bent at a 45-degree angle; then immediately explode your body skyward and back up into the high plank position.

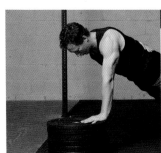

ASSIST

Place your hand on a plyo box, a stack of weight plates, or a yoga brick before trying this one flat on the ground. Increasing the incline decreases the difficulty.

DIP TO L-SIT

The Dip to L-Sit targets your triceps and your core like no other exercise. This movement is best done on a set of plyo boxes, but tall parallettes, dip bars, or two benches will also work.

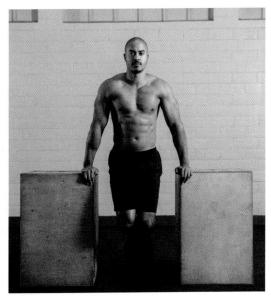

[1] Position yourself between two plyo boxes placed shoulder width apart. Place your hands on the front edges of the boxes, and use your arms to push your body up and off the ground while raising your legs up and swinging your feet behind you as you hold them together tightly. Keep your shoulders down and pushed away from your ears.

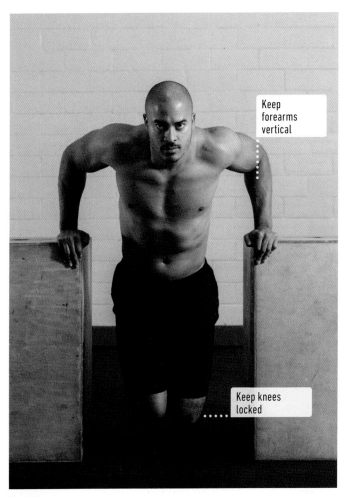

Keep forearms vertical

Keep knees locked

[2] Drop into a dip by bending your arms and lowering your body until your shoulders are slightly below your elbows.

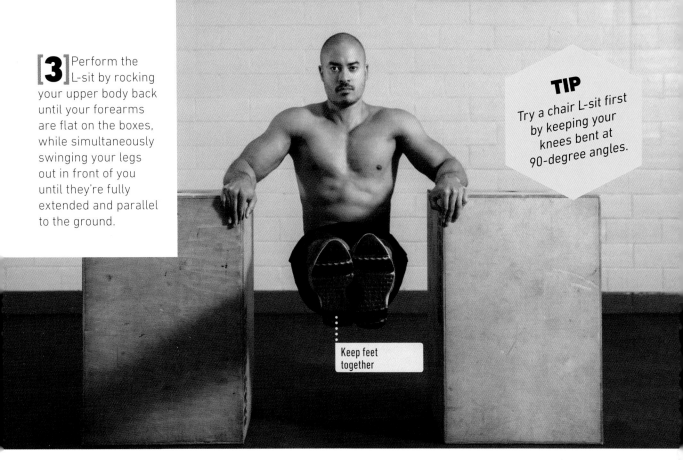

[3] Perform the L-sit by rocking your upper body back until your forearms are flat on the boxes, while simultaneously swinging your legs out in front of you until they're fully extended and parallel to the ground.

TIP
Try a chair L-sit first by keeping your knees bent at 90-degree angles.

Keep feet together

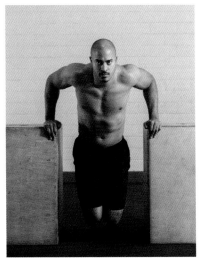

[4] Rock your upper body forward and swing your legs back behind you to return the dip position.

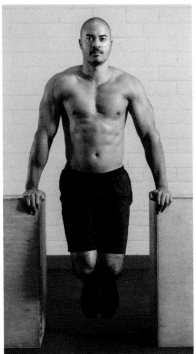

[5] Straighten your arms to push your body up and back into the starting position.

MASTERING THE MOVEMENT

GOOD: 1 set of 4
BETTER: 2 sets of 6
MASTERED: 3 sets of 8

TRIPLE-CLAP PUSH-UP

The Triple-Clap Push-Up requires exceptional coordination, hand speed, flexibility, and explosiveness. It's an uncommon feat of strength, but it's one you can accomplish with practice.

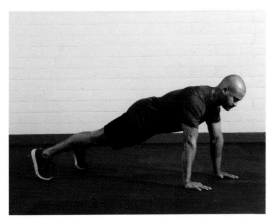

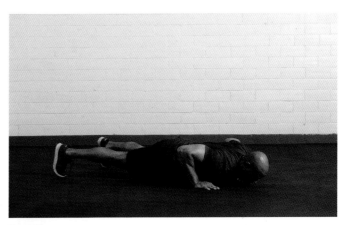

[1] Begin in a high plank position with your arms locked, your hands positioned slightly wider than shoulder width apart, and your fingers pointing forward. Push your shoulders down and away from your ears, and keep your abs and glutes tight.

[2] Slowly drop into a low push-up position, until your chest is just above the floor and your elbows are bent at 45-degree angles.

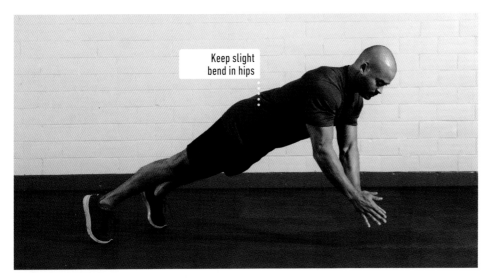

Keep slight bend in hips

[3] Explosively push your torso away from the ground, and immediately perform a front clap as you ascend.

[4] Immediately perform a clap behind your back at the apex of the movement.

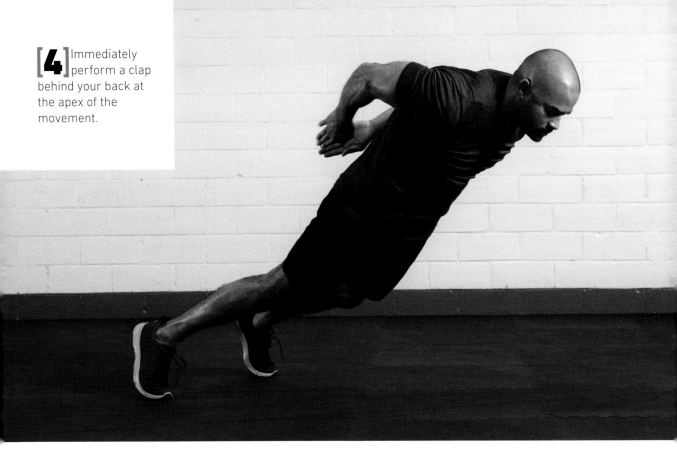

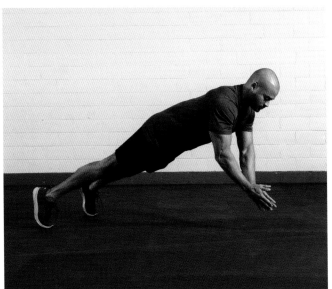

[5] Immediately perform a second front clap as you begin to descend.

MASTERING THE MOVEMENT

GOOD: 1 set of 2
BETTER: 2 sets of 3
MASTERED: 3 sets of 5

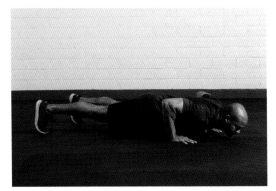

[6] Return your hands to the ground to land softly in a low push-up position.

CRUCIFIX PUSH-UP

The Crucifix Push-Up demands exceptional shoulder and core strength and engages your entire upper body. The arm positioning makes this movement a significant challenge.

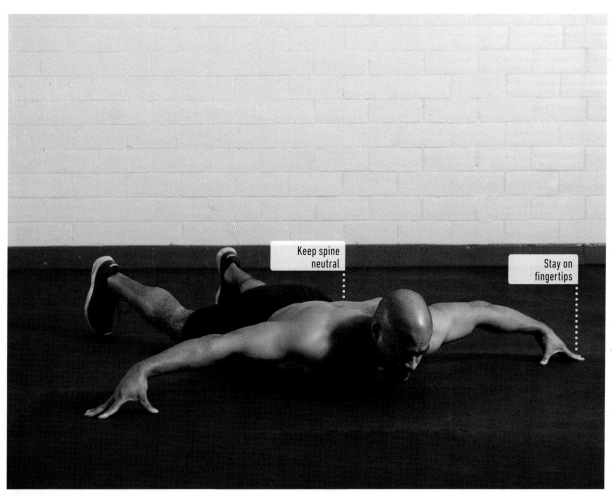

Keep spine neutral

Stay on fingertips

[1] Begin in a prone position on the ground with your legs extended behind you and your arms extended away from your shoulders. Keep your spine neutral and face your eyes to the ground. Press your fingertips into the ground, and rotate your shoulders so your elbows are facing up.

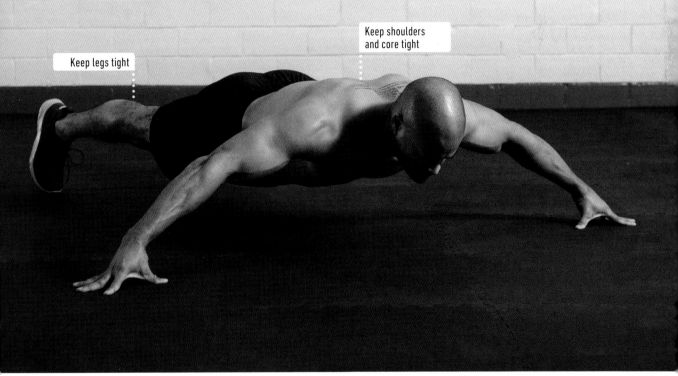

Keep legs tight

Keep shoulders
and core tight

MASTERING THE MOVEMENT

GOOD: 1 set of 3
BETTER: 2 sets of 4
MASTERED: 3 sets of 5

[2] Squeeze your glutes and engage your core, inhale deeply, then press your toes and fingertips into the ground to lift your entire body off the ground as a single unit. Exhale sharply as you descend back to the ground.

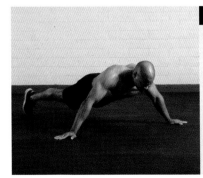

ASSIST

Perform with your hands placed flat on the ground and positioned slightly closer to your shoulders.

HANDSTAND PUSH-UP

The Handstand Push-Up builds impressive upper-body strength and power. This one may seem daunting at first, but your confidence will grow as you master the basics.

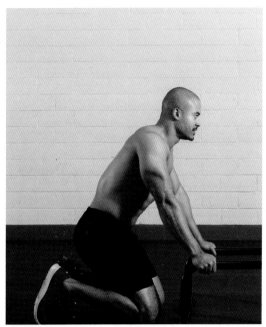

[1] Place a set of paralettes shoulder width apart in front of you. Begin in a kneeling position with your hands positioned on the front of the paralettes.

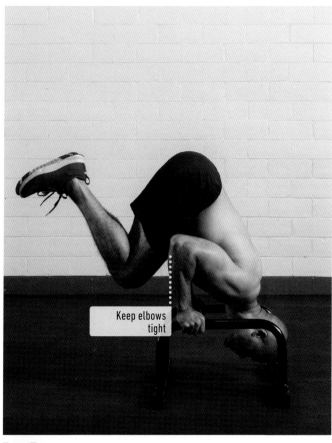

Keep elbows tight

[2] Slowly roll your body forward as you lower your head toward the ground, keeping your glutes and core tight to stabilize your movement. Continue rolling until you've completely shifted your weight to your hands and your feet are off the ground.

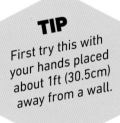

TIP
First try this with your hands placed about 1ft (30.5cm) away from a wall.

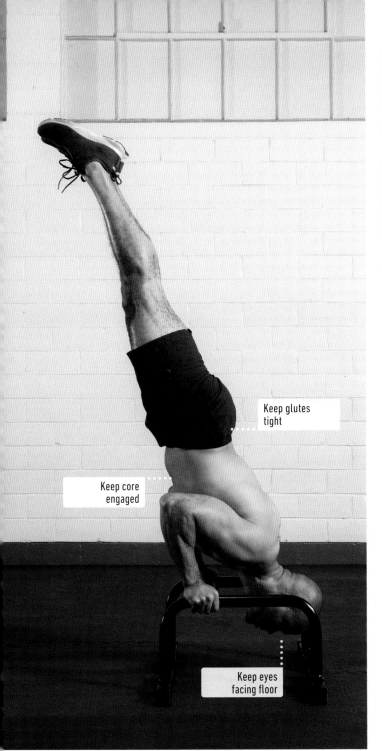

Keep glutes
tight

Keep core
engaged

Keep eyes
facing floor

[3] Fully extend your legs vertically, keeping your body at a slight angle.

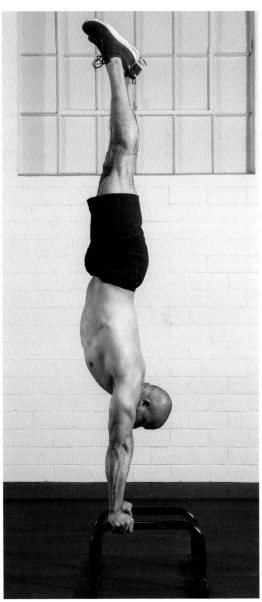

[4] Press through your hands to slowly push your body into a fully extended vertical position.

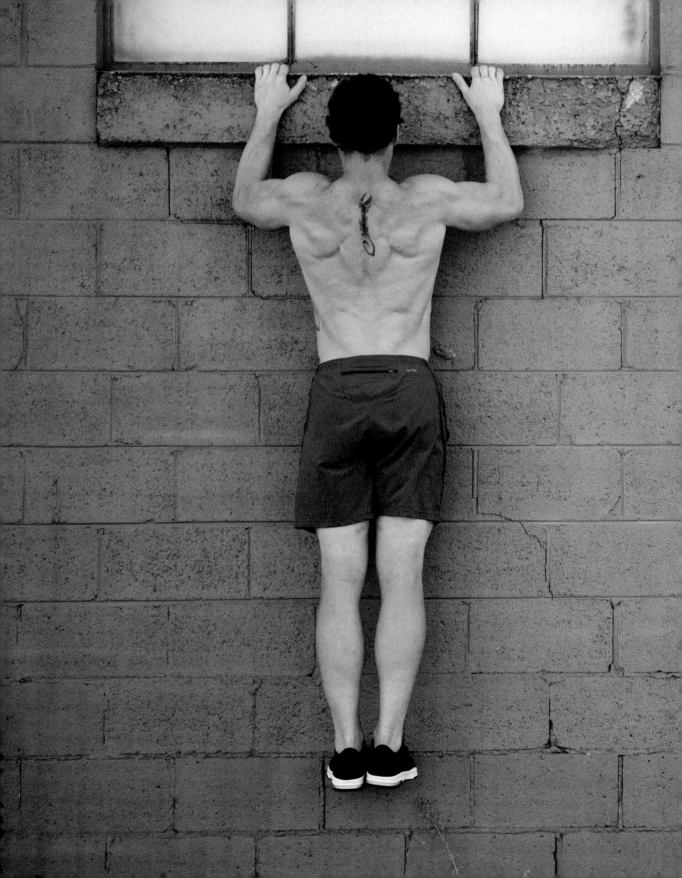

BODYWEIGHT ROW

The Bodyweight Row will build a strong back, which is imperative for building a rock-solid physique, by working your lats, traps, and biceps, as well as the stabilizer muscles in between.

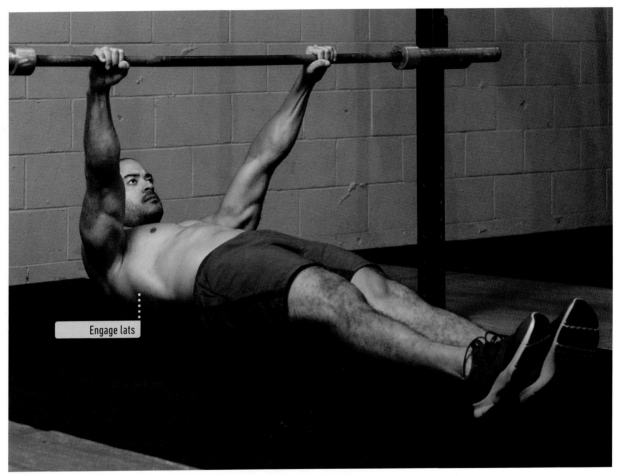

Engage lats

[1] Lie on your back underneath a racked bar that is positioned just above where you can reach it with extended arms. Grasp the bar with an overhand grip, and your hands placed slightly wider than shoulder width apart. Fully extend your legs in front of you with your shoulders, hips, knees, and ankles all aligned to form an inverted plank position.

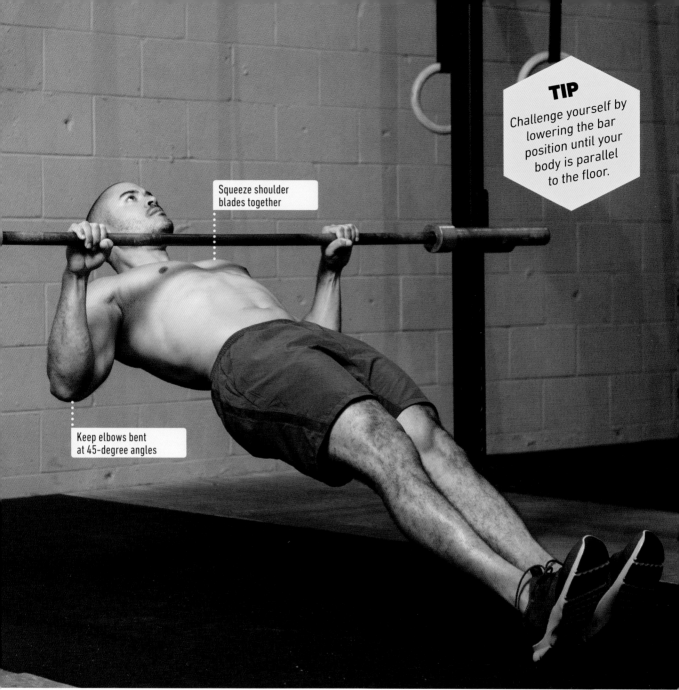

Squeeze shoulder blades together

Keep elbows bent at 45-degree angles

TIP
Challenge yourself by lowering the bar position until your body is parallel to the floor.

[2] Engage your core and pull yourself up until your chest touches the bar, and then slowly lower yourself back down to the starting position.

MASTERING THE MOVEMENT

GOOD: 2 sets of 3
BETTER 2: 3 sets of 10
MASTERED: 3 sets of 20

CHIN-UP

The Chin-Up will build strength in your shoulders, arms, and core. While a Pull-Up utilizes an overhand grip, the Chin-Up utilizes an underhand grip to better target the biceps.

[1] Begin in a dead-hang position by grasping the bar with an underhand grip, with your hands positioned slightly wider than shoulder width apart and your elbows locked.

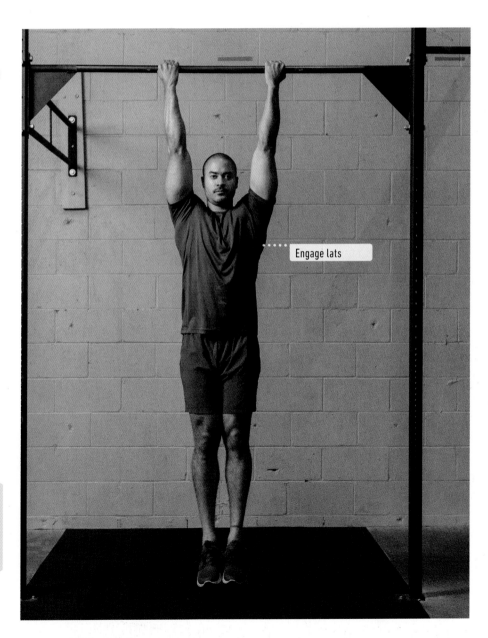

Engage lats

TIP
Execute every rep with full range of motion to maximize benefits.

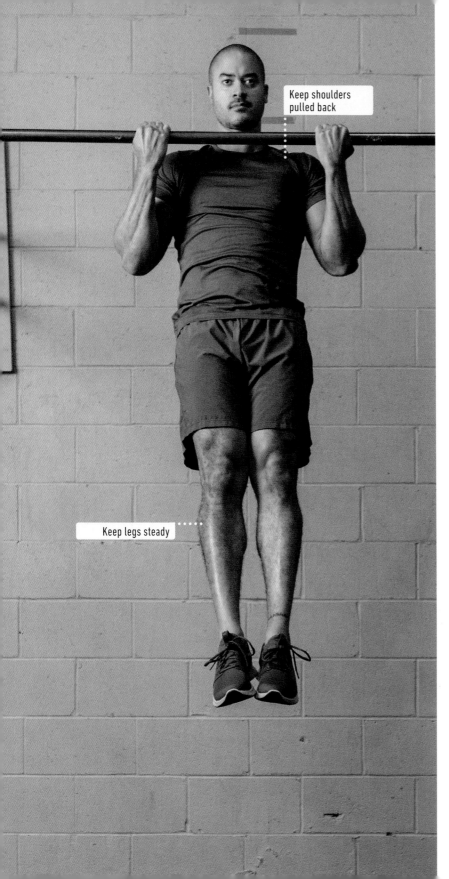

Keep shoulders
pulled back

Keep legs steady

[2] Squeeze your glutes and engage your core as you pull your body up until your chin clears the bar. Pause, and then slowly lower yourself back down to the dead-hang position.

MASTERING THE MOVEMENT

GOOD: 1 set of 5
BETTER: 2 sets of 10
MASTERED: 3 sets of 12

PULL-UP

The Pull-Up is one of the most difficult pulling exercises to execute, but once you have it mastered, you'll see your upper-body strength advance to previously unknown levels.

[1] Begin in a dead-hang position by grasping the bar with an overhand grip, with your hands positioned slightly wider than shoulder width apart and your elbows locked.

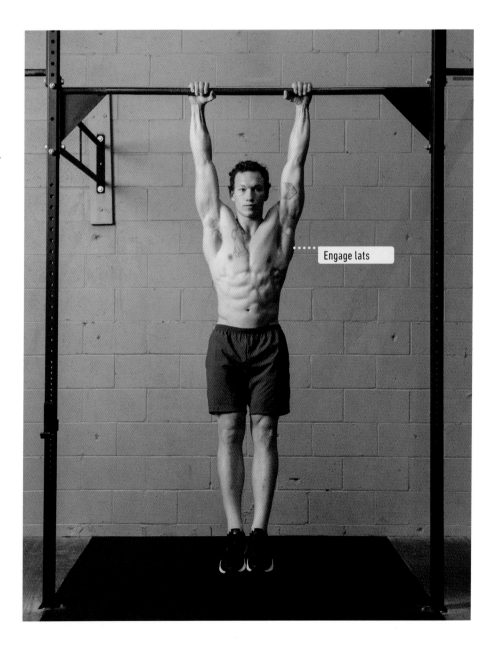

Engage lats

[2] Exhale forcefully, squeeze your glutes, and tightly engage your core as you pull your body up until your chin clears the bar. Pause, and then slowly lower yourself back down into a dead-hang position, inhaling as you descend.

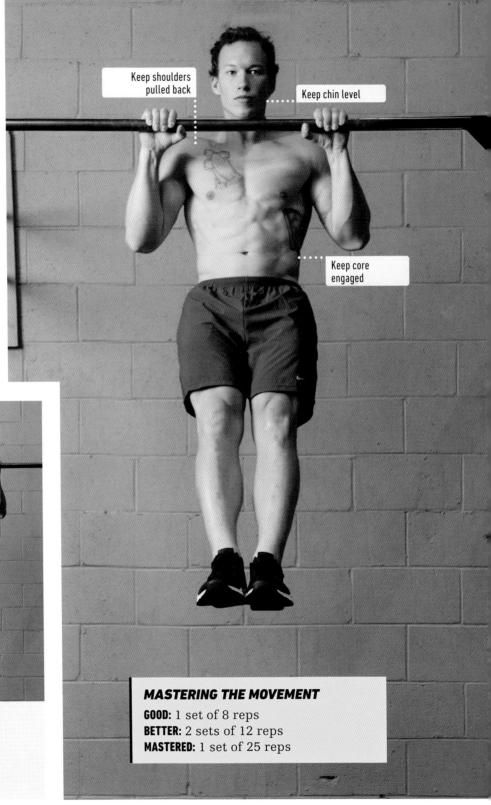

Keep shoulders pulled back

Keep chin level

Keep core engaged

ASSIST

Place one foot in a band that is secured around the bar; progressively use lighter bands as your strength improves.

MASTERING THE MOVEMENT

GOOD: 1 set of 8 reps
BETTER: 2 sets of 12 reps
MASTERED: 1 set of 25 reps

WEIGHTED PULL-UP

The Weighted Pull-Up requires all the raw power and grit you can muster to pull extra weight over the bar, but you'll be rewarded with exponential gains in upper-body strength.

[1] Place a dumbbell between your thighs and cross your legs to secure. Begin in a dead-hang position by grasping the bar with an overhand grip with your hands positioned slightly wider than shoulder width apart, and your elbows locked.

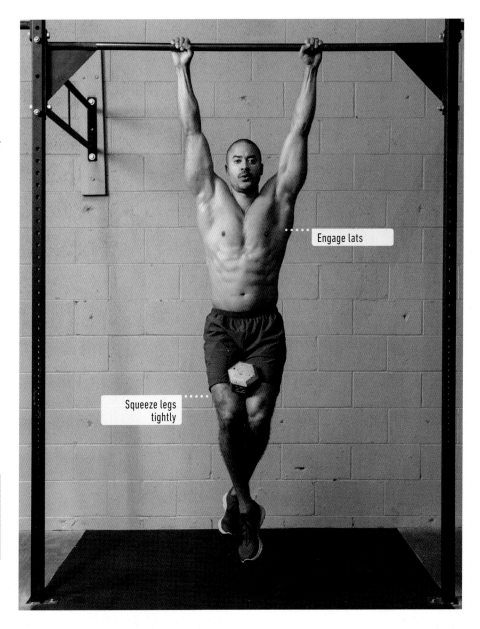

Engage lats

Squeeze legs tightly

TIP
You can also use a weighted belt or ankle weights.

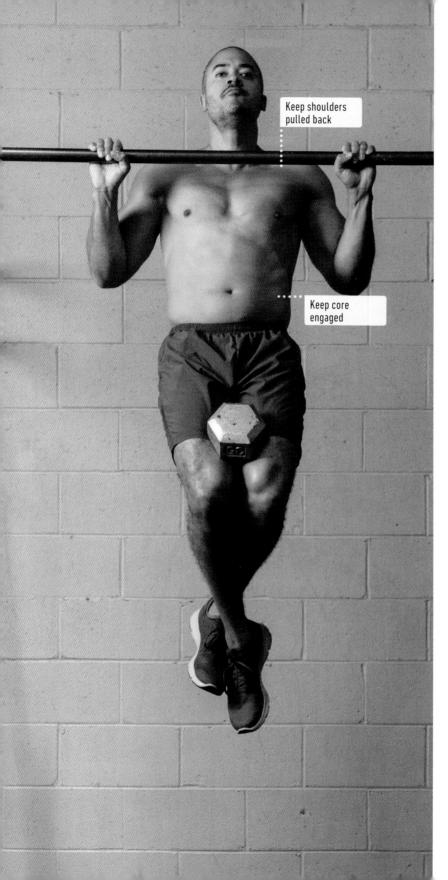

Keep shoulders pulled back

Keep core engaged

[2] Squeeze your glutes, tightly engage your core, and exhale forcefully as you pull your body up until your chin clears the bar. Pause, and then slowly lower yourself down and back into a dead-hang position, inhaling as you descend.

MASTERING THE MOVEMENT

GOOD: 1 set of 3
BETTER: 2 sets of 5
MASTERED: 3 sets of 8

COMMANDO PULL-UP

The Commando Pull-Up is even tougher than it looks and requires engaging your entire upper body to prevent twisting. It's tough, but it will build brutal upper-body strength.

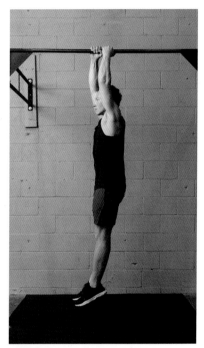

[1] Begin in a dead-hang position with your elbows locked and your hands stacked side by side, using opposing overhand grips on each side of the bar.

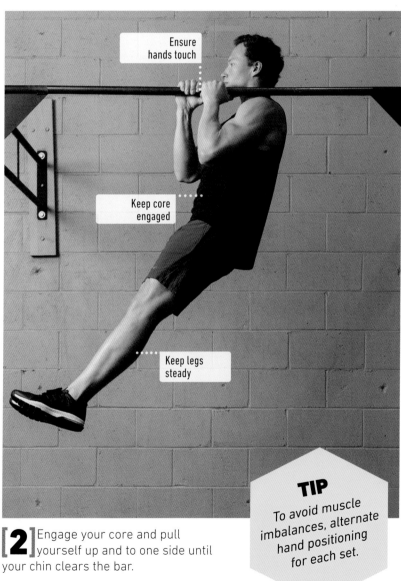

Ensure hands touch

Keep core engaged

Keep legs steady

[2] Engage your core and pull yourself up and to one side until your chin clears the bar.

TIP
To avoid muscle imbalances, alternate hand positioning for each set.

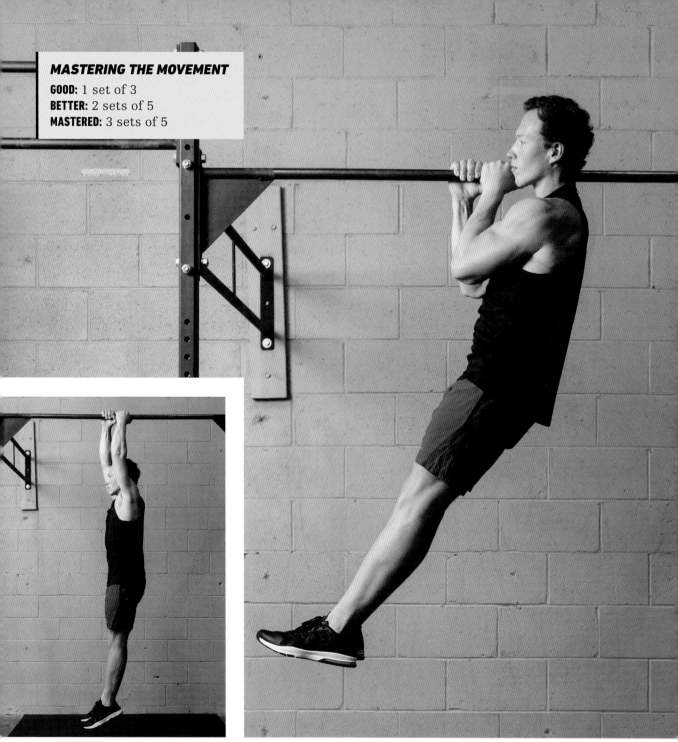

[3] Lower yourself back down into a dead-hang position.

[4] Pull your body back up again until your chin clears the bar, this time moving your head to the opposite side of the bar.

IN-AND-OUT GRIP PULL-UP

The In-and-Out Grip Pull-Up combines two grips in one dynamic plyo exercise to work your back and biceps. The narrow grip targets your arms, while the wide grip targets your lats.

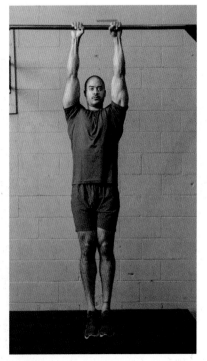

[1] Begin in a dead-hang position by grasping the bar with an overhand grip with your hands positioned slightly narrower than shoulder width apart, and your elbows locked.

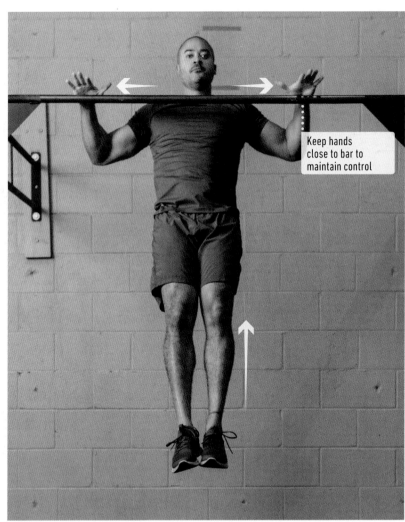

Keep hands close to bar to maintain control

[2] With force and speed and in one fluid motion, pull your body up until your chin clears the bar while simultaneously sliding your hands out to a wide-grip position.

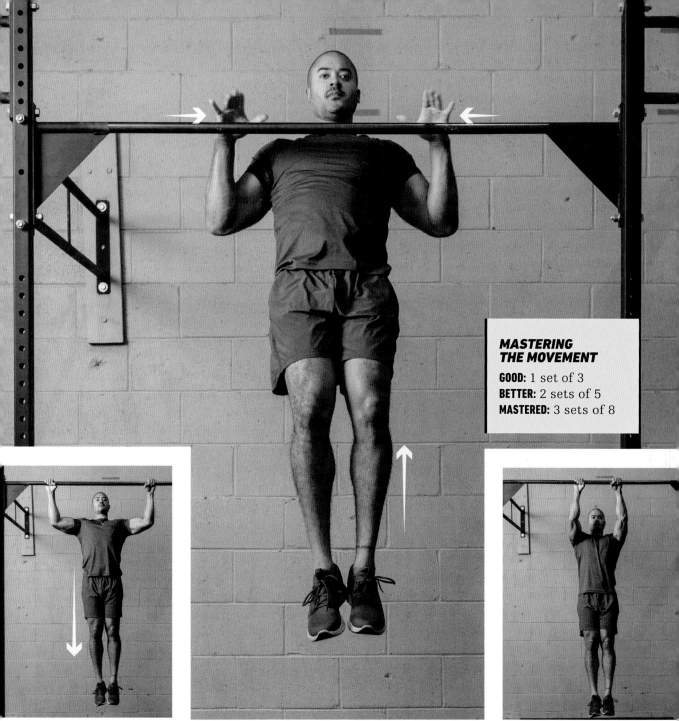

MASTERING THE MOVEMENT

GOOD: 1 set of 3
BETTER: 2 sets of 5
MASTERED: 3 sets of 8

[3] Slowly lower your body down until your arms are fully extended and you're back in a dead-hang position.

[4] With force and speed and in one fluid motion, pull your body back up until your chin clears the bar while simultaneously sliding your hands back into a narrow-grip position.

[5] Slowly lower your body back down until your arms are fully extended and you're back in a dead-hang position.

UNEVEN-GRIP PULL-UP

In addition to creating exceptional raw pulling power in your shoulders, lats, and arms, the Uneven-Grip Pull-Up will build awesome strength in your hands and fingers.

[1] Begin in a modified dead-hang position by looping a rolled towel over a pull-up bar and using a hammer grip to grasp the towel at the bottom as tightly as possible. Grasp the bar with your opposite hand using an overhand grip. Your hands should be positioned shoulder-width apart.

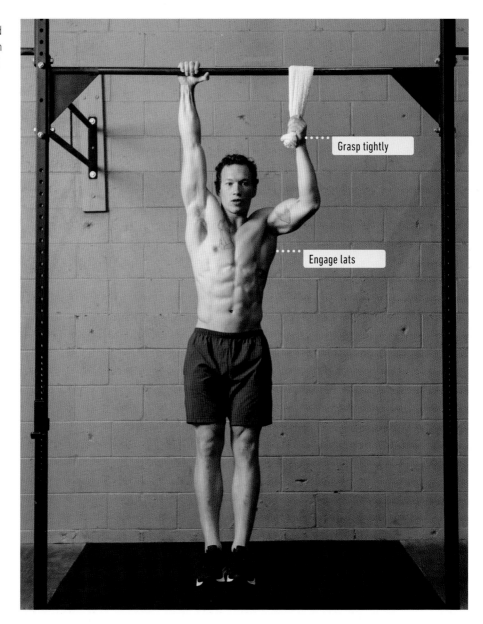

Grasp tightly

Engage lats

[2] Initiate an upward movement by pulling with your higher hand first, and at the halfway point, pulling down on the towel with your lower hand until your chin clears the bar. Pause at the top position before slowly lowering back down into the modified dead-hang position.

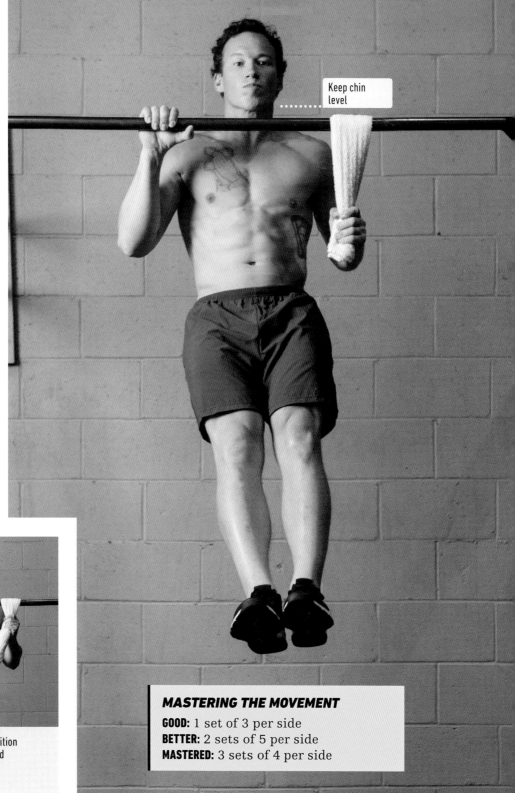

Keep chin level

ASSIST

Start with a narrower hand position with your lower hand positioned higher on the towel.

MASTERING THE MOVEMENT
GOOD: 1 set of 3 per side
BETTER: 2 sets of 5 per side
MASTERED: 3 sets of 4 per side

ARCHER PULL-UP

The Archer Pull-Up adds a significantly higher degree of resistance to a traditional Pull-Up and is also a good intermediate step toward executing the One-Arm Pull-Up.

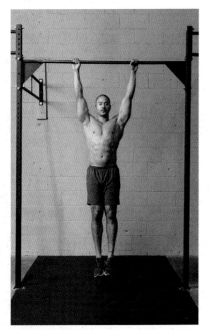

[1] Begin in a dead-hang position with your hands placed in an overhand grip and positioned slightly wider than shoulder width apart on the bar.

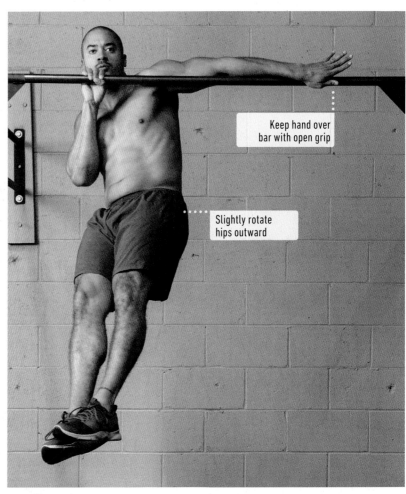

Keep hand over bar with open grip

Slightly rotate hips outward

[2] Engage your lats and drive your elbow down to pull your body up and to the right side of the bar, while simultaneously extending your left arm across the bar and pushing down with your left hand.

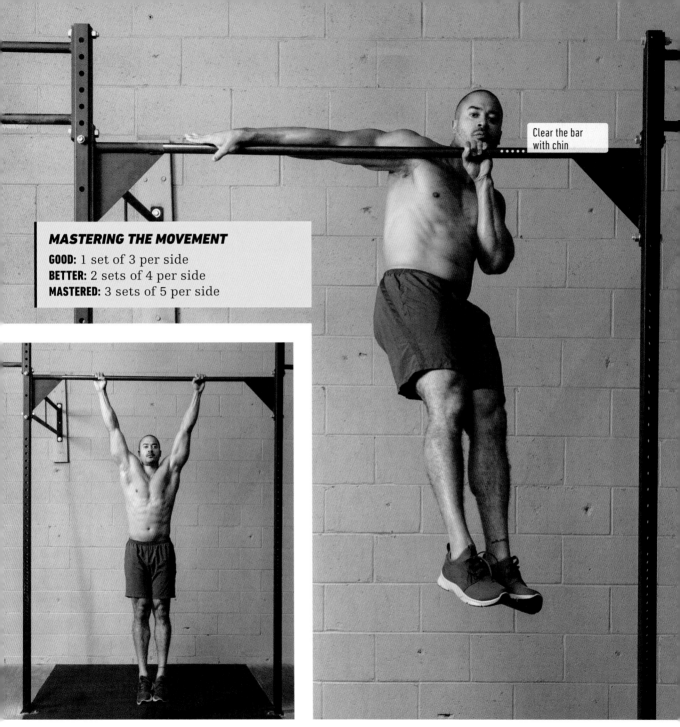

Clear the bar with chin

MASTERING THE MOVEMENT

GOOD: 1 set of 3 per side
BETTER: 2 sets of 4 per side
MASTERED: 3 sets of 5 per side

[3] Slowly lower your body back down into a dead-hang position.

[4] Engage your lats and drive your elbow down to pull your body up and to the left side of the bar, while simultaneously extending your right arm across the bar and pushing down with your right hand.

CLAPPING PULL-UP

While most pull-ups are performed slowly, the Clapping Pull-Up requires speed, control, and explosive power to gain the height necessary to clap your hands in midair.

[1] Begin in a dead-hang position by grasping the bar with an overhand grip, with your hands positioned slightly wider than shoulder width apart and your elbows locked.

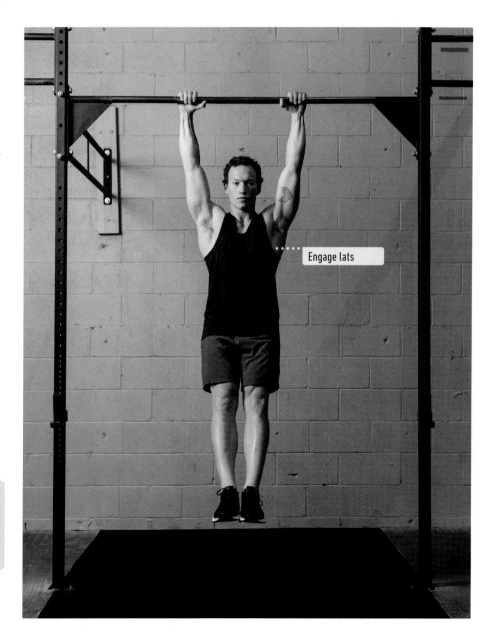

Engage lats

TIP
To avoid damaged shoulders, keep your lats engaged at all times.

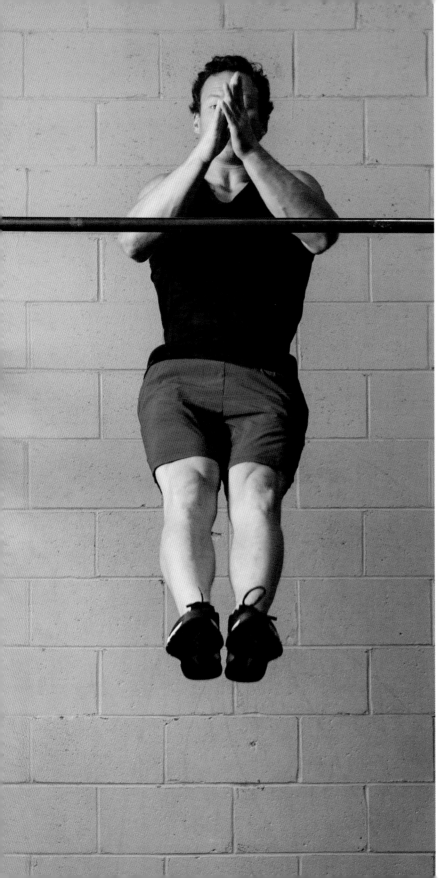

[2] Exhale forcefully, and in one fluid motion explosively pull yourself up as fast and as high as possible while simultaneously performing a clap at the top of the movement; then then immediately place your hands back on the bar to catch yourself as you descend. Slowly lower your body back down into a dead-hang position.

MASTERING THE MOVEMENT

GOOD: 1 set of 2
BETTER: 2 sets of 3
MASTERED: 3 sets of 4

MUSCLE-UP

The Muscle-Up works nearly every muscle in your upper body. To execute it you'll need explosive pulling power to get over the bar and superior strength to push yourself above it.

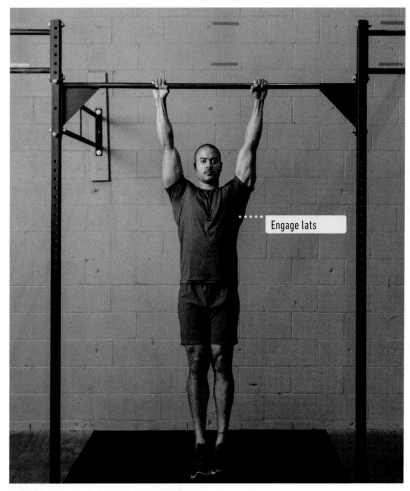

Engage lats

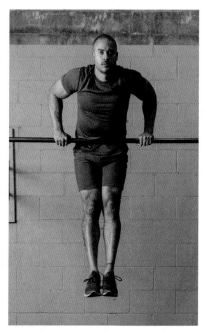

[1] Begin in a dead-hang position by grasping the bar with an overhand grip, with your hands positioned slightly wider than shoulder width apart and your elbows locked.

[2] Exhale forcefully, squeeze your glutes, and tightly engage your core as you pull yourself up until your hips are level with the bar. Pause.

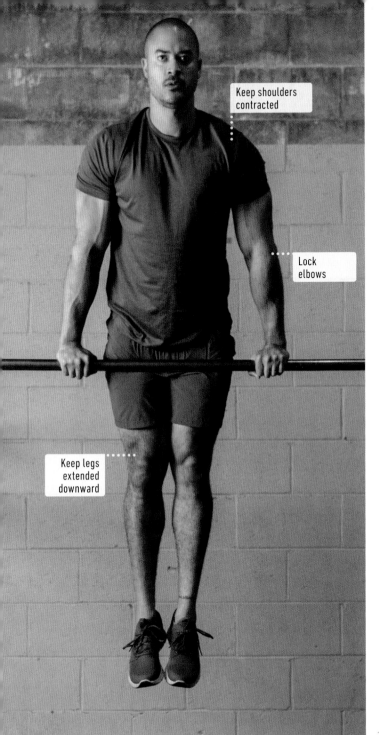

Keep shoulders contracted

Lock elbows

Keep legs extended downward

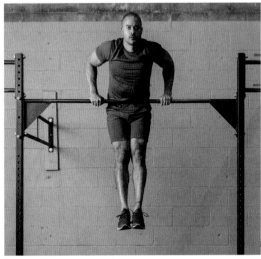

[4] Slowly lower your body back down until your hips are level with the bar. Pause.

[3] Extend your elbows to push yourself straight up and into a full tricep extension. Pause.

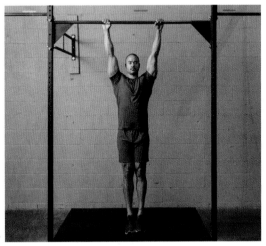

[5] Slowly lower yourself down and back into a dead-hang position.

L-SIT ROPE CLIMB

A basic rope climb is an excellent movement for building upper-body strength in your arms and core, but adding an L-sit to the climb takes the challenge to an entirely different level.

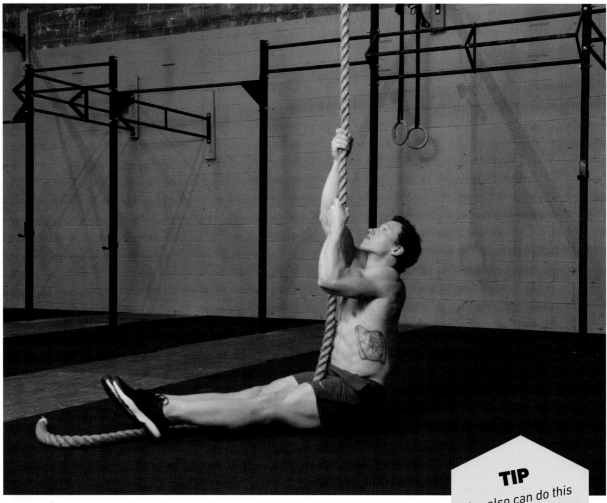

[1] Begin in a seated position on the ground with your legs extended and a rope placed between your legs. Grasp the rope tightly, with both hands placed in a hand-over-hand position.

TIP
You also can do this on a short rope looped over a pull-up bar.

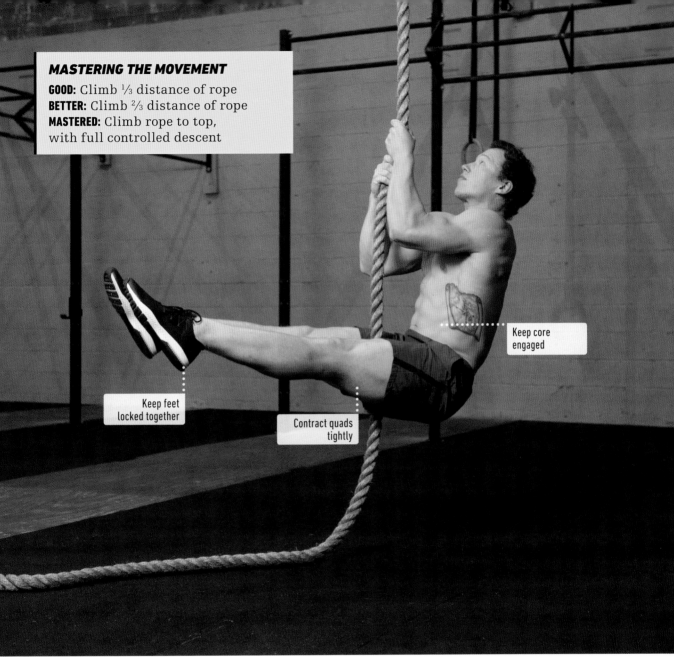

MASTERING THE MOVEMENT

GOOD: Climb ⅓ distance of rope
BETTER: Climb ⅔ distance of rope
MASTERED: Climb rope to top,
with full controlled descent

Keep core
engaged

Keep feet
locked together

Contract quads
tightly

[2] Begin pulling yourself up the rope, hand over hand, with your legs extended and your core engaged, until you reach the top of the rope, and then slightly bend your knees, and slowly lower yourself back to the ground.

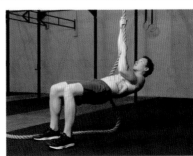

ASSIST

Keep your feet flat on the ground as you use your arms to climb the rope. You can also bend your knees as you climb, and place your feet on the rope to brake your body as you descend.

ONE-ARM PULL-UP

The One-Arm Pull-Up requires tremendous power and focus to execute and is a movement that very few people have achieved, but with perseverance and practice, you'll nail it.

[1] Begin in a dead-hang position with one hand placed on the bar in an overhand grip position, and the opposite arm extended out to your side.

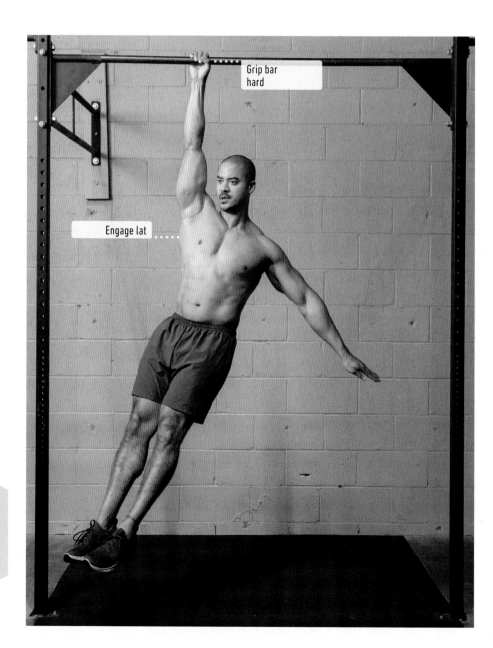

Grip bar hard

Engage lat

TIP
To avoid injury, attempt only after you can perform 15 pull-ups.

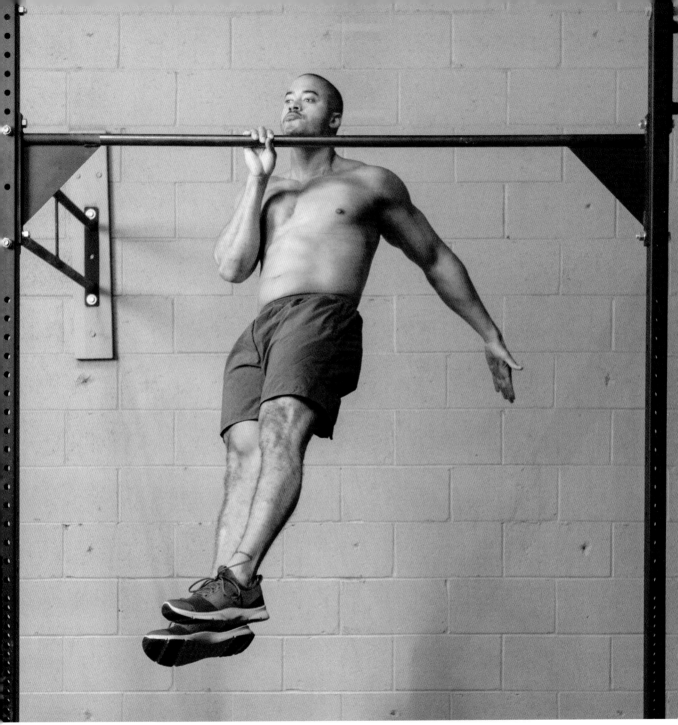

[2] Fully engage your lat and oblique, and slightly rotate your hips inward toward your working arm to begin pulling yourself up. As you near the top, turn your elbow in and pull down as forcefully as possible to bring your chin up and over the bar.

MASTERING THE MOVEMENT

GOOD: 1 set of 1 per side
BETTER: 1 set of 2 per side
MASTERED: 1 set of 3 per side

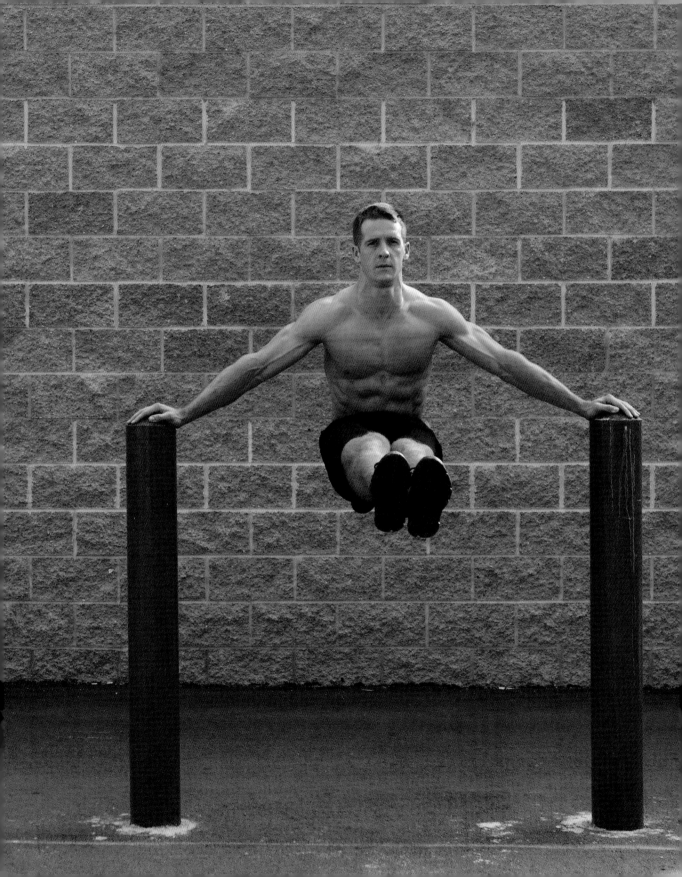

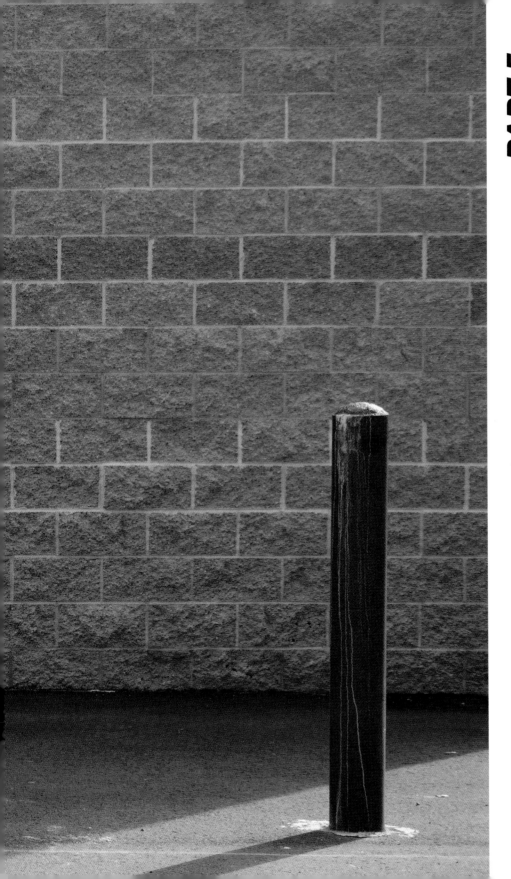

PART 5
CORE MOVEMENTS

HANGING KNEE RAISE

The Hanging Knee Raise targets your lower abdominals, hip flexors, and lower back, and increases stability in your upper back and shoulders. It's simple, but it builds serious core strength.

[1] Begin in a dead-hang position by grasping the bar with an overhand grip with your hands positioned slightly wider than shoulder width apart and your elbows locked.

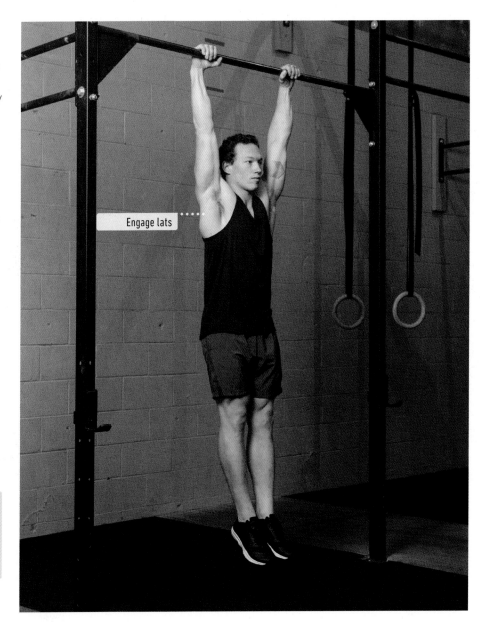

Engage lats

TIP
Don't jerk your legs up, and avoid swinging back and forth.

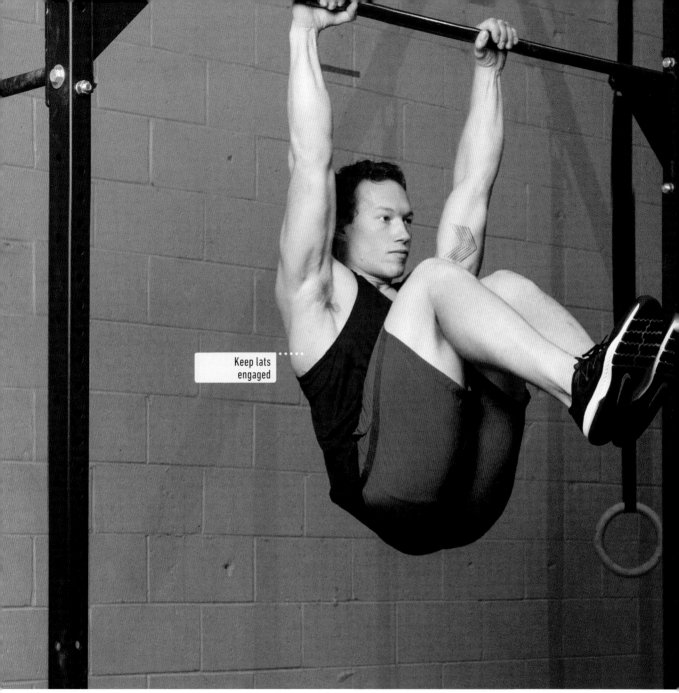

Keep lats engaged

[2] Engage your core, and use your abdominal muscles to curl your hips forward as you pull your knees up to your shoulders. Pause when your knees reach your chest, and then slowly return to the dead-hang position.

MASTERING THE MOVEMENT

GOOD: 1 set of 5
BETTER: 2 sets of 10
MASTERED: 3 sets of 20

OBLIQUE STARFISH

The Oblique Starfish will help prepare you for the Human Flag. It engages your shoulders, triceps, quads, and all of the stabilizer muscles of your core, particularly your obliques.

[1] Begin in a high plank position with your arms locked, your hands positioned slightly narrower than shoulder width apart, and your fingers pointing forward. Push your shoulders down and away from your ears, and keep your abs and glutes tight.

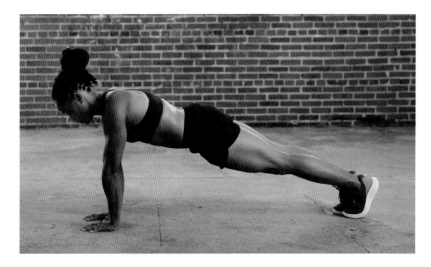

[2] In one fluid motion, slowly swing your left arm out, while rolling your legs and hips up until your hand is pointing skyward and you're resting on the outside of your right foot.

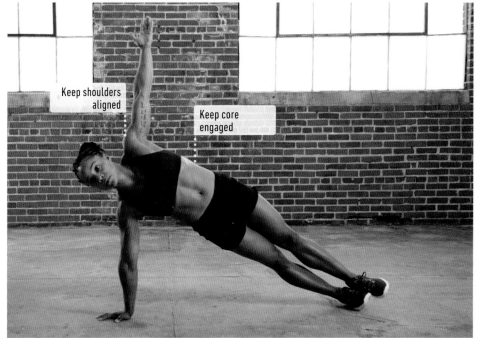

Keep shoulders aligned

Keep core engaged

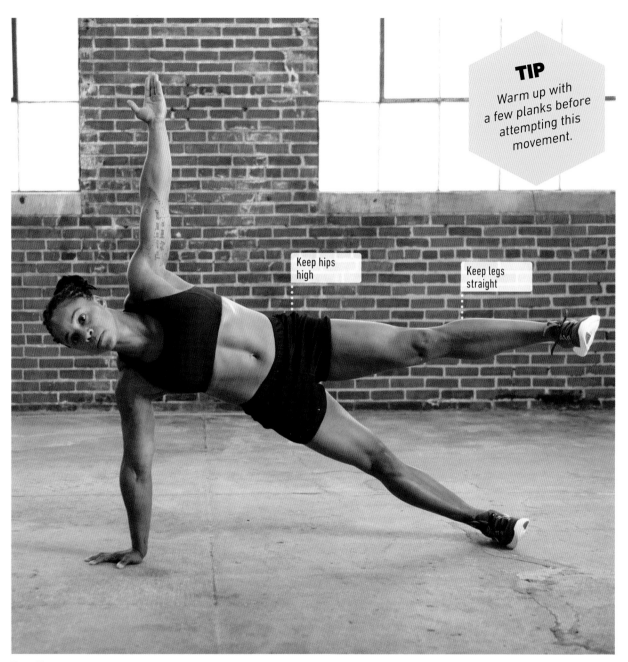

Keep hips high

Keep legs straight

TIP
Warm up with a few planks before attempting this movement.

[3] Keeping both feet flexed, lift your left leg into the air and then bring your legs back together before lowering your arm back down and rolling your body back into a high plank position. Repeat on the opposite side.

MASTERING THE MOVEMENT

GOOD: hold 15 seconds per side
BETTER: hold 30 seconds per side
MASTERED: hold 1 minute per side

HANGING LEG RAISE

The Hanging Leg Raise will work nearly every muscle group in your body and will help stabilize your core by strengthening the muscles that surround your vital organs.

[1] Begin in a dead-hang position by grasping the bar with an overhand grip and positioning your hands slightly wider than shoulder width apart. Lock your elbows, engage your lats and core, and keep your shoulders pushed down and away from your ears. Extend your legs slightly forward.

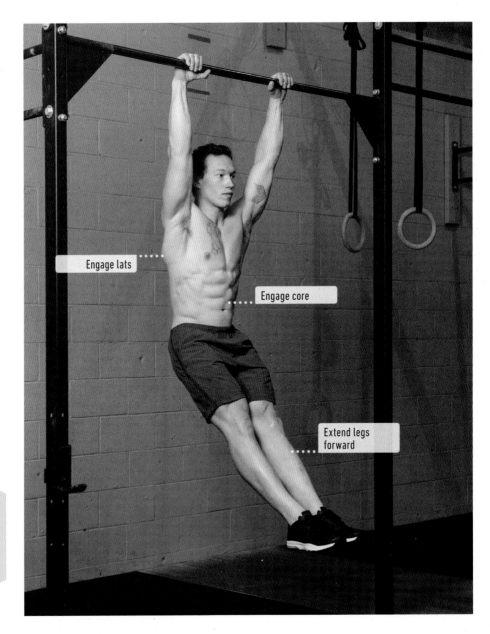

Engage lats

Engage core

Extend legs forward

TIP
Don't swing your body, and control your speed.

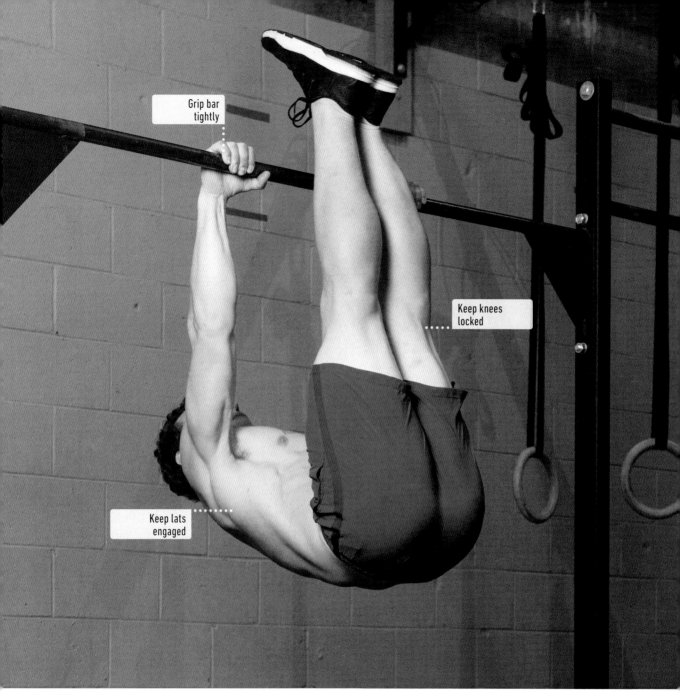

Grip bar
tightly

Keep knees
locked

Keep lats
engaged

[2] Engage your abdominal muscles to raise your legs up until they're completely vertical. Pause, and then slowly lower your legs back down to the starting position.

MASTERING THE MOVEMENT

GOOD: 1 set of 5
BETTER: 2 sets of 10
MASTERED: 3 sets of 12

L-SIT

It's hard to beat the L-Sit for building whole-body strength and control. To pull this one off, your shoulders, arms, and core all have to remain solid, and your legs flexible and strong.

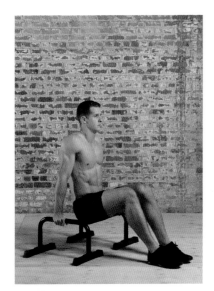

[1] Position a pair of paralettes shoulder width apart on the ground. Begin in an elevated sitting position with your hands centered on the grips. Push yourself up until your elbows are locked and your shoulders are pushed down and away from your ears. Bend your knees, and keep your feet flat on the ground.

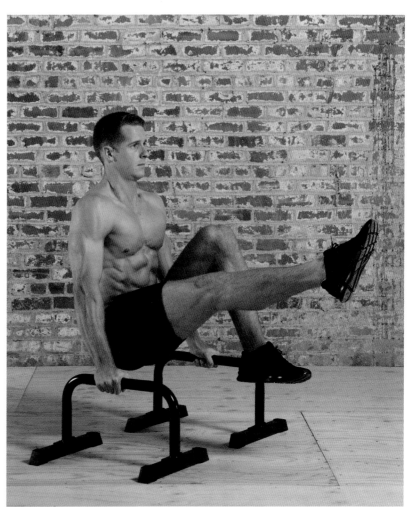

[2] Bring both knees up into a tuck position at your chest and then fully extend one leg in front of you.

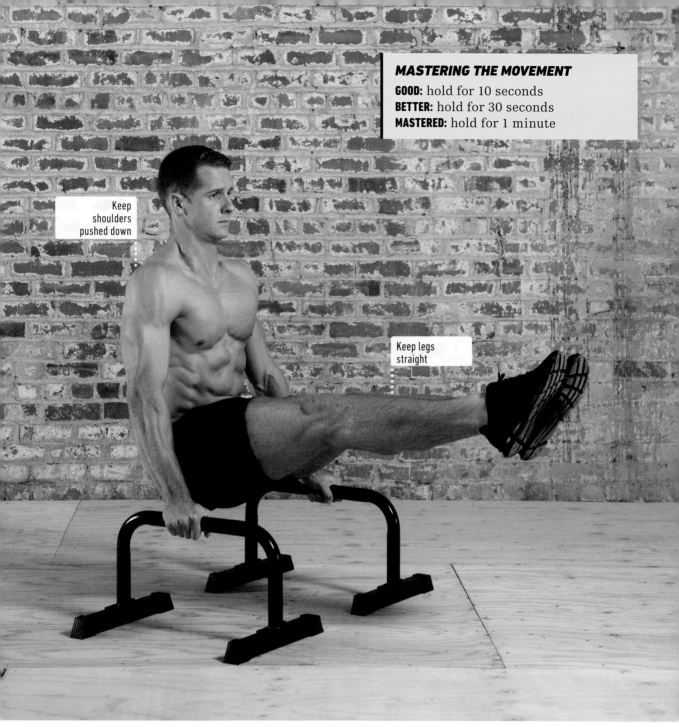

MASTERING THE MOVEMENT
GOOD: hold for 10 seconds
BETTER: hold for 30 seconds
MASTERED: hold for 1 minute

Keep
shoulders
pushed down

Keep legs
straight

[3] Extend the opposite leg out in front of you
until both legs are fully extended.

AB-CRUNCH SHREDDER

A cross between a Hanging Knee Raise and a Dragon Flag, the Ab-Crunch Shredder dynamically engages your core and arms to build power and stability in your core.

[1] Grasp the bar using an overhand grip with your hands positioned shoulder width apart. Engage your lats to pull yourself up until your arms are flexed at 90-degree angles. Engage your core and extend your legs slightly out front of you. Point your toes forward.

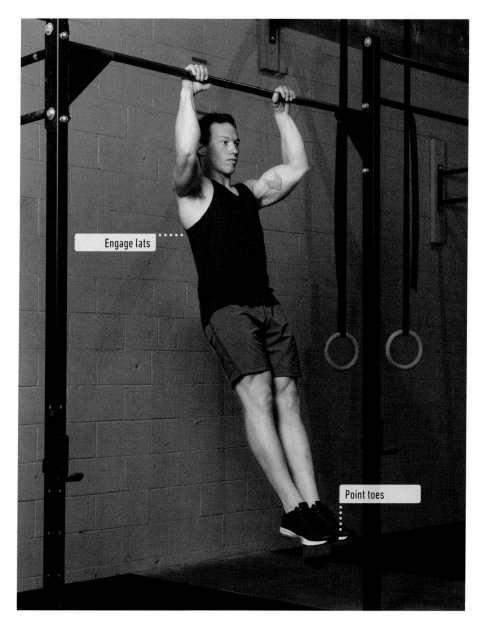

Engage lats

Point toes

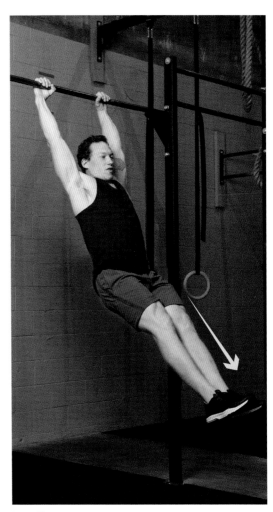

[2] Load your body into a hanging tuck position by engaging your abdominals, and then pulling your knees up as high as possible to your chest.

[3] Extend your arms as you kick your legs out at a 45-degree angle; then immediately retract your arms and legs back into the hanging tuck position. Repeat the movement in a rapid-fire back-and-forth motion.

BUZZSAW

The Buzzsaw uses the upper body, as well as hip flexion and extension, to really shred your core. Elevating your hips vertically helps target your lower abs.

[1] Place a folded towel on a smooth, slick surface. Lower yourself into a flat position on your stomach with your toes resting on the towel and your hands and arms extended directly in front of you.

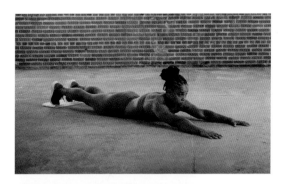

[2] Keeping your head and back straight, pull through your forearms and hinge at your elbows to slide your feet forward, and push your body up into a plank position.

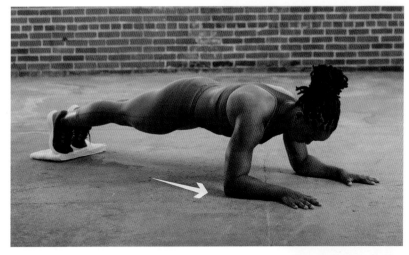

[3] Push through your hands to slide your feet, and pull your body forward and into a low push-up position.

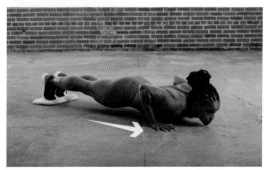

[4] Push down into the floor to rise up into a high plank position.

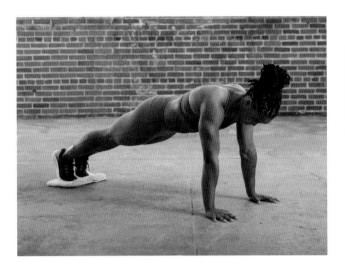

TIP
You can wear socks or use exercise sliders if you don't have a towel.

[5] Engage your glutes and abs to slide your feet forward and push your hips skyward while simultaneously rising up onto your toes. Complete the movement by returning to the high plank position.

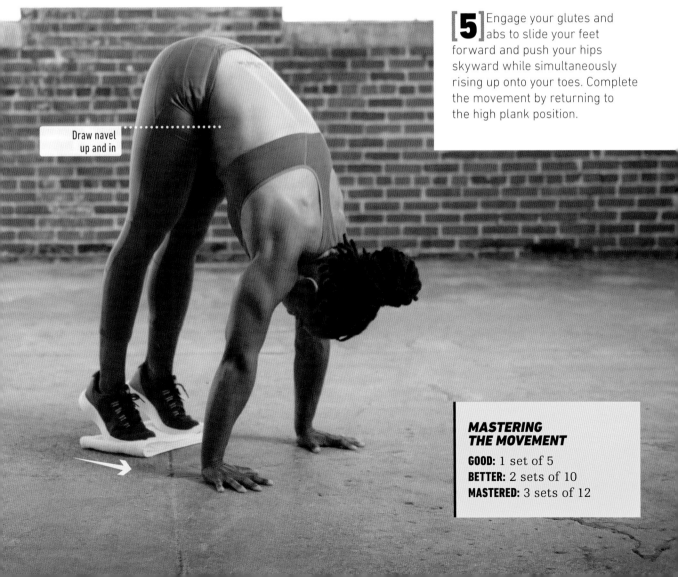

Draw navel up and in

MASTERING THE MOVEMENT

GOOD: 1 set of 5
BETTER: 2 sets of 10
MASTERED: 3 sets of 12

HEADSTAND LEG RAISE

The Headstand Leg Raise strengthens the lower back, develops total body strength and balance, promotes body control and awareness, and is good training for more advanced moves.

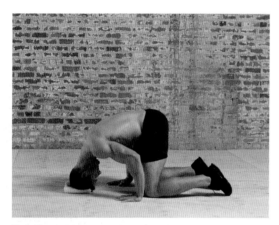

[1] Kneel in front of a folded towel. Place your hands flat on the ground, positioned shoulder width apart and just beyond your knees. Tuck your chin to your chest, and place your head on the towel.

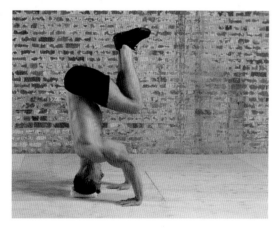

[2] Slowly begin rolling forward, transferring your weight to your hands and head, until your body is stacked with your hips above your head.

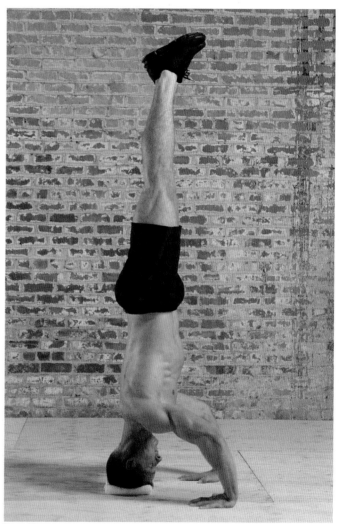

[3] Keeping your core engaged, extend your toes, squeeze your glutes, and tighten your quads to slowly extend your legs up until they are fully vertical.

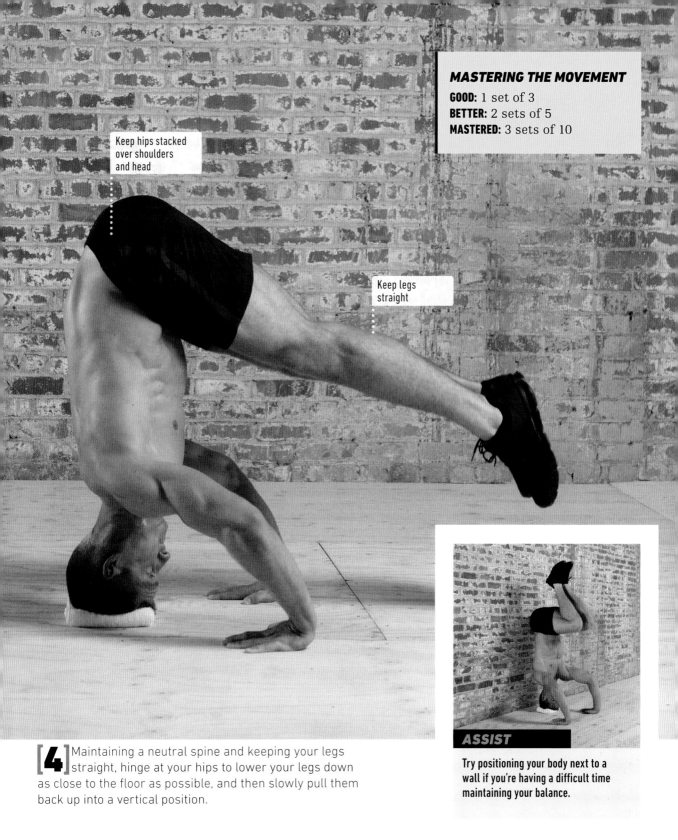

Keep hips stacked
over shoulders
and head

MASTERING THE MOVEMENT
GOOD: 1 set of 3
BETTER: 2 sets of 5
MASTERED: 3 sets of 10

Keep legs
straight

[4] Maintaining a neutral spine and keeping your legs straight, hinge at your hips to lower your legs down as close to the floor as possible, and then slowly pull them back up into a vertical position.

ASSIST

Try positioning your body next to a wall if you're having a difficult time maintaining your balance.

DRAGON FLAG

Everyone wants a six pack, and the Dragon Flag will make it happen by engaging your entire core and hammering your abs. It also helps keep your torso strong and upright when you walk.

[1] Begin by lying flat on your back and grasping a bar or other sturdy object behind your head with opposing overhand grips. Engage your abdominals to bring your legs up until they're stacked directly over your hips.

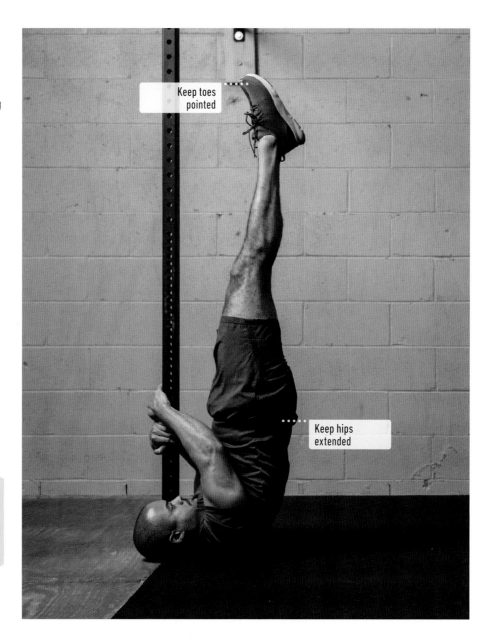

Keep toes pointed

Keep hips extended

TIP
Keep your abs, lower back, and glutes constantly engaged.

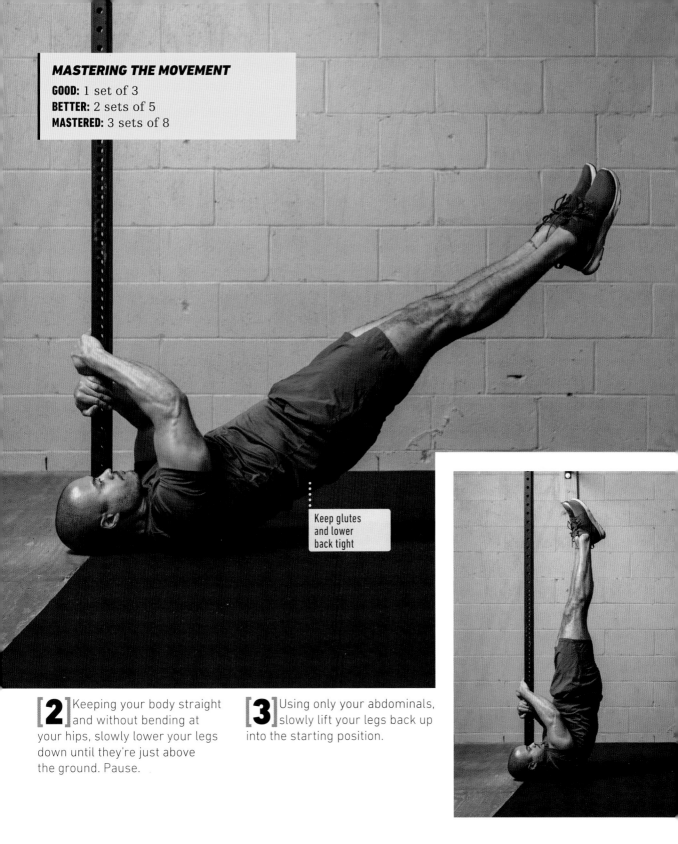

Keep glutes
and lower
back tight

[2] Keeping your body straight and without bending at your hips, slowly lower your legs down until they're just above the ground. Pause.

[3] Using only your abdominals, slowly lift your legs back up into the starting position.

TUCK LEVER

The Tuck Lever works your core, builds strength in your shoulders and lats, and develops your grip strength—all important elements for progressing to the Front Lever.

[1] Begin in a dead-hang position by grasping the bar with an overhand grip, with your hands positioned slightly wider than shoulder width apart and your arms fully extended.

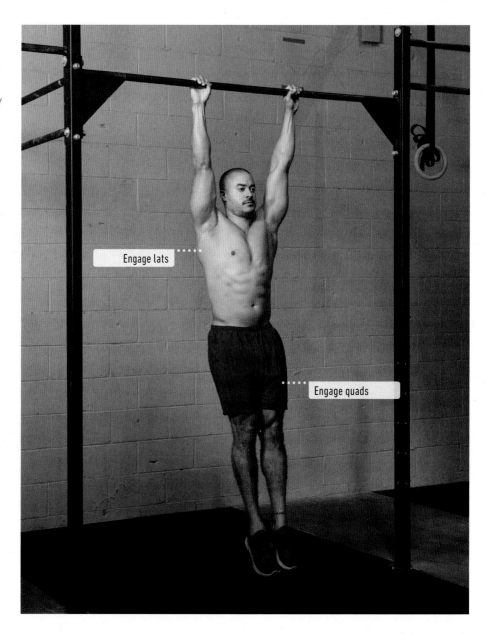

Engage lats

Engage quads

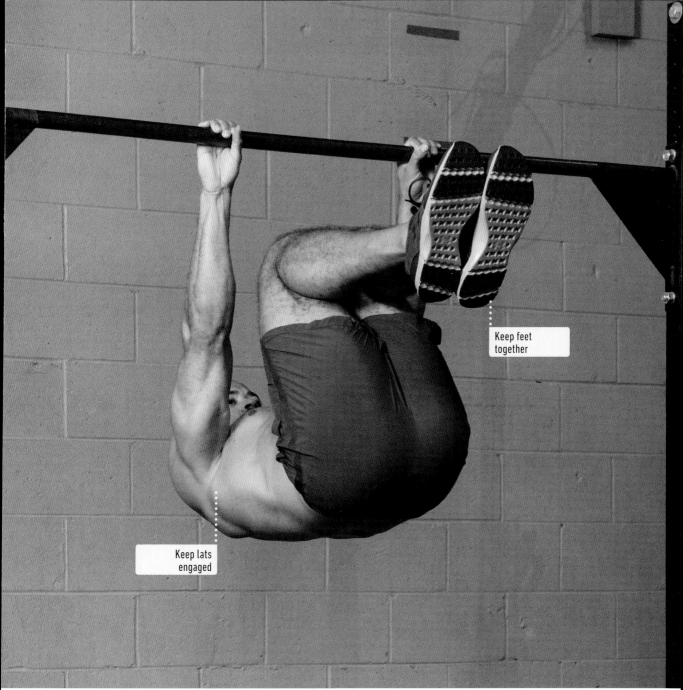

Keep feet together

Keep lats engaged

[2] Engage your abdominals to pull your hips up and draw your knees in toward your chest, while allowing your body to roll back until your torso is parallel to the ground. Hold for as long as possible before slowly rolling back into a dead-hang position.

MASTERING THE MOVEMENT

GOOD: hold for 3 seconds
BETTER: hold for 5 seconds
MASTERED: hold for 10+ seconds

FRONT LEVER

The Front Lever takes the Tuck Lever to the next level to strengthen the entire body. Don't be intimidated by this one—you can develop the necessary skills to master it.

[1] Begin in a dead-hang position by grasping the bar with an overhand grip, with your hands positioned slightly wider than shoulder width apart and your arms fully extended.

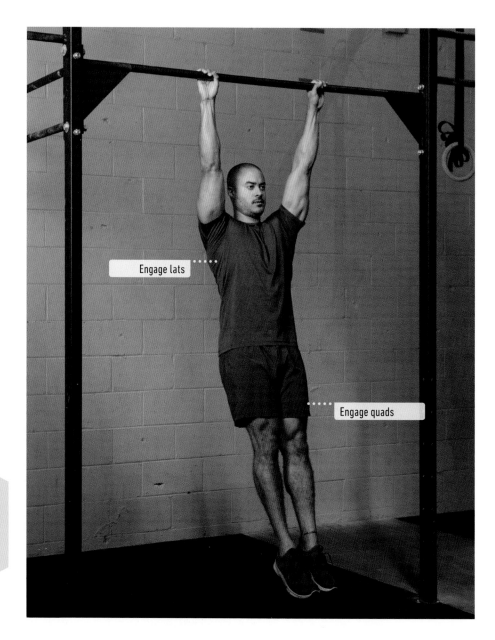

Engage lats

Engage quads

TIP
Keep your glutes, quads, and calves engaged through the entire movement.

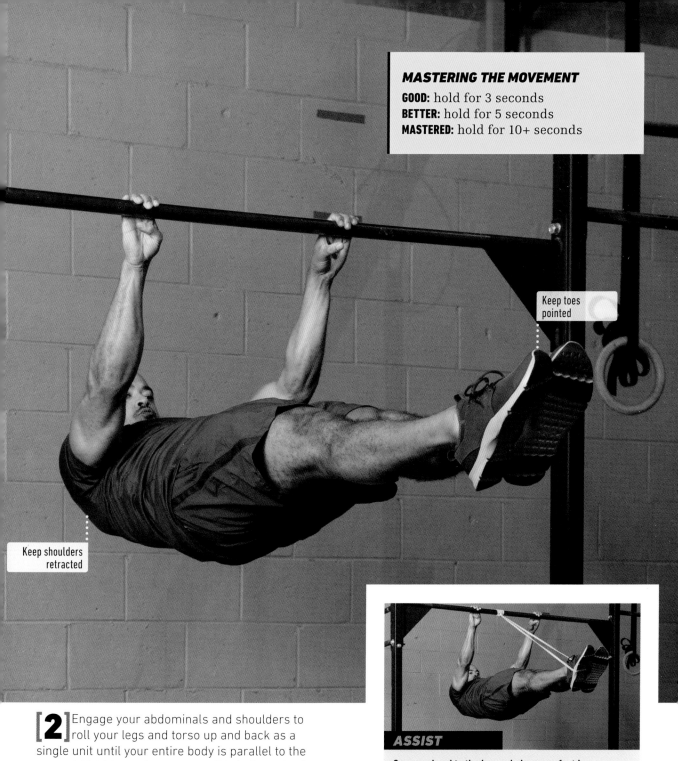

Keep toes pointed

Keep shoulders retracted

[2] Engage your abdominals and shoulders to roll your legs and torso up and back as a single unit until your entire body is parallel to the ground. Hold for as long as possible before slowly rotating back into a dead-hang position.

ASSIST

Secure a band to the bar and place one foot in the band. You can progressively use lighter bands as your strength increases.

TUCK HUMAN FLAG

The Tuck Human Flag takes patience to master and requires significant strength and body awareness to execute, but it will build a solid core as well as rock hard delts and lats.

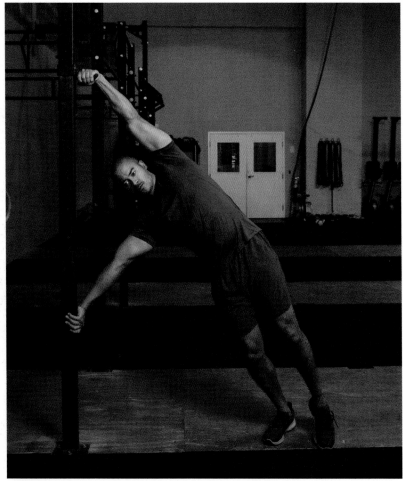

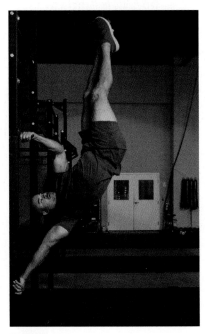

TIP

Since the outside arm will be the most engaged, use your strongest arm on top.

[1] Stand just far enough from a vertical pole that you can stretch your outside arm over your body to grasp the pole as high as possible with an overhand grip. Using an underhand grip, grasp the pole as low as possible with your inside hand. Your hands should be positioned as wide as possible, and both feet should remain in contact with the ground.

[2] Keeping both arms straight, forcefully push into the pole with your lower arm while simultaneously pulling as hard as possible with your upper arm to pull your legs and torso up into a vertical flag position.

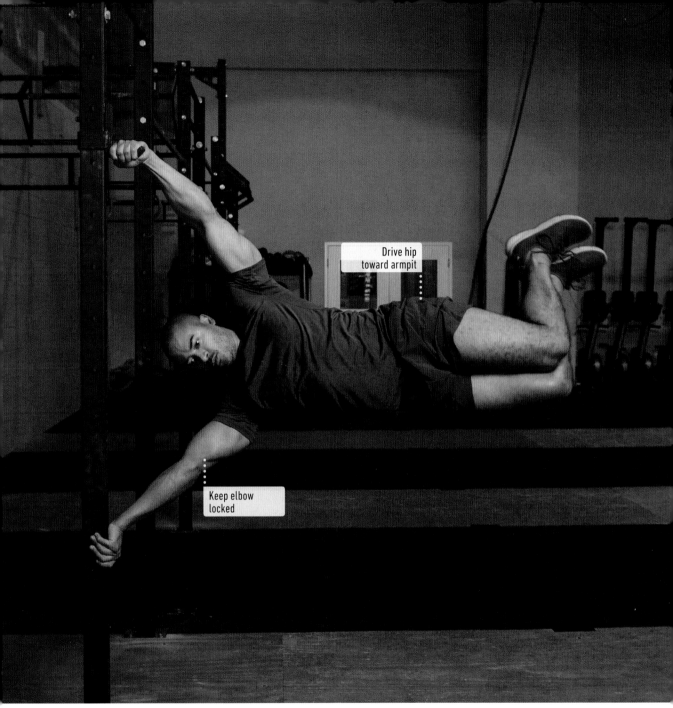

Drive hip
toward armpit

Keep elbow
locked

[3] Begin bending your knees as you slowly lower your legs and torso down until your body is parallel to the ground. Hold.

MASTERING THE MOVEMENT

GOOD: hold for 3 seconds
BETTER: hold for 5 seconds
MASTERED: hold for 10+ seconds

HUMAN FLAG

The Human Flag is the ultimate full-body movement and requires an an exceptional blend of strength, stability, and control. If you've made it this far, it's time to get after this!

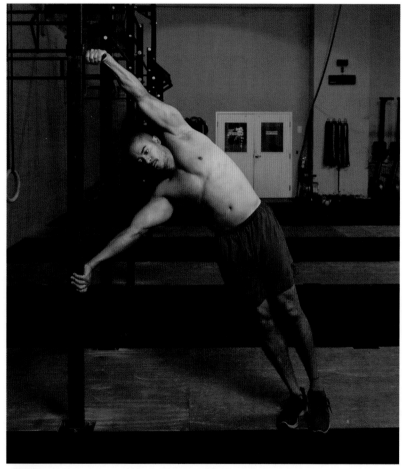

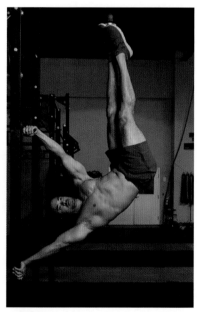

TIP
Train by first rising into the vertical flag only, and holding for as long as possible.

[1] Stand just far enough from a vertical pole that you can stretch your outside arm over your body to grasp the pole as high as possible with an overhand grip. Using an underhand grip, grasp the pole as low as possible with your inside hand. Your hands should be positioned as wide as possible, and both feet should still remain on the ground.

[2] Keeping both arms straight, forcefully push into the pole with your lower arm while simultaneously pulling as hard as possible with your upper arm to pull your legs and torso up into a vertical flag position.

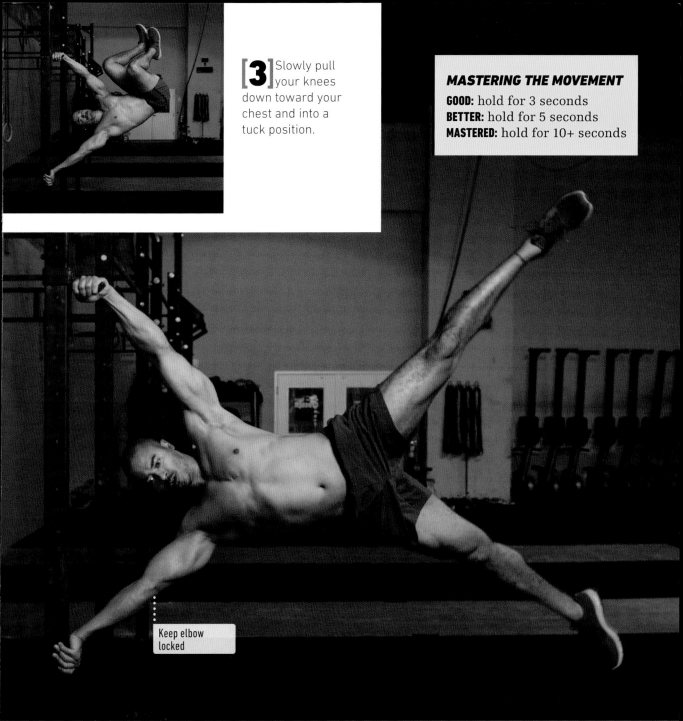

[3] Slowly pull your knees down toward your chest and into a tuck position.

MASTERING THE MOVEMENT

GOOD: hold for 3 seconds
BETTER: hold for 5 seconds
MASTERED: hold for 10+ seconds

Keep elbow locked

[4] Slowly lower your torso while simultaneously extending your legs out until your torso is parallel to the ground and your legs are fully extended in an open flag position. Hold.

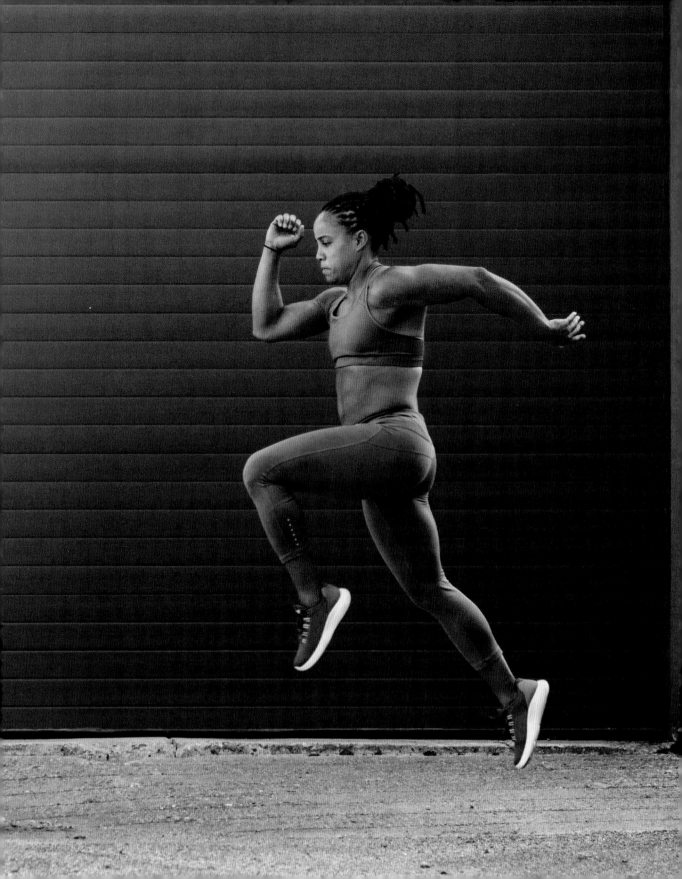

PART 6
CARDIO MOVEMENTS

HALF BURPEE

Similar to the Burpee but without the jump and the push-up, the Half Burpee will get your heart pumping, improve your core stability, and increase your hip and ankle mobility.

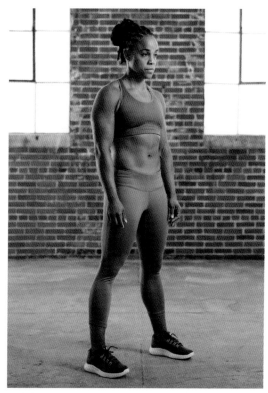

[1] Begin in a standing position with your arms at your sides and your feet placed slightly wider than shoulder width apart.

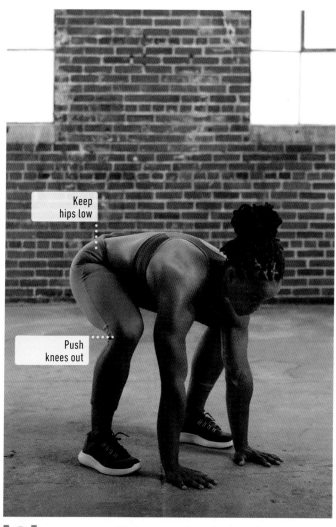

Keep hips low

Push knees out

[2] Lower yourself into a squat position and place your hands flat on the ground.

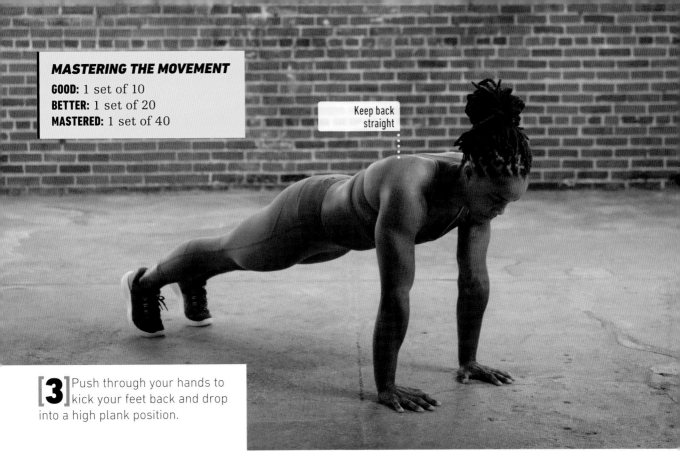

Keep back straight

[3] Push through your hands to kick your feet back and drop into a high plank position.

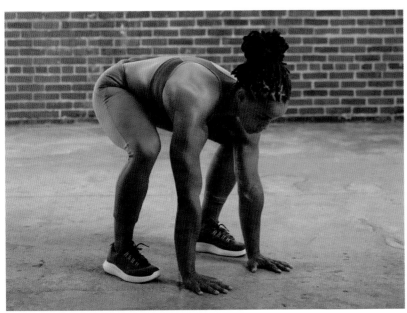

[4] Jump your feet forward and back into the squat position.

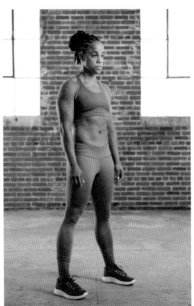

[5] Stand back up into the starting position.

SKATER

The Skater will build strength, stability, and explosive power in your legs by targeting your hips and quads. It's an outstanding movement for burning fat and developing agility.

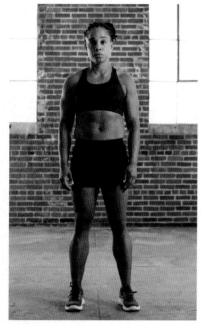

[1] Begin in a standing position with your arms at your sides, your feet positioned shoulder width apart, and your knees slightly bent.

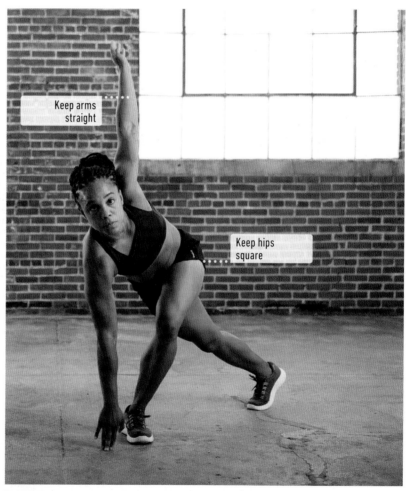

Keep arms straight

Keep hips square

[2] Extend your left leg behind you while simultaneously swinging your left arm up and behind you and reaching your right arm down to the ground.

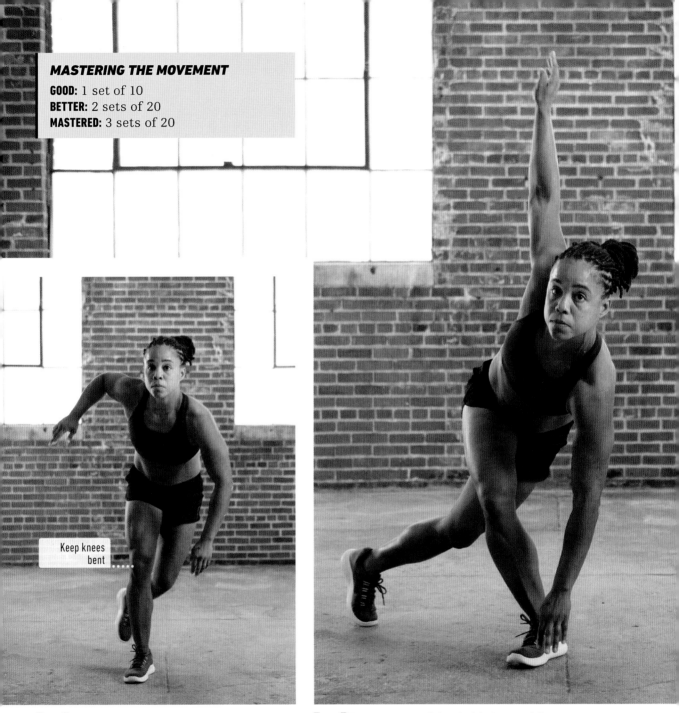

Keep knees bent

[3] In a motion similar to that of a speed skater, swing your arms and push from your left foot to launch over to the opposite side and land on your right foot.

[4] Extend your left leg behind you while simultaneously swinging your right arm up and behind you and reaching your left arm down to the ground. Repeat from side to side in a rapid, controlled fashion.

180 ROCKET JUMP

The 180 Rocket Jump conditions the heart and targets the hip musculature, which is crucial for stabilization as you pivot and move through athletic movements.

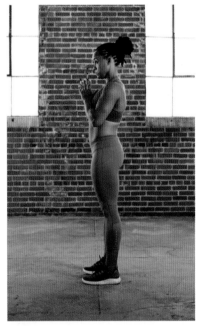

[1] Begin in an athletic stance with your feet positioned slightly wider than your hips and your hands pressed together in front of your chest.

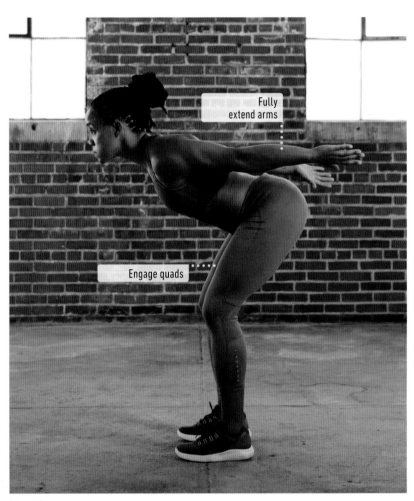

Fully extend arms

Engage quads

[2] Load your body by dropping into a deep squat and quickly swinging your arms down and behind you.

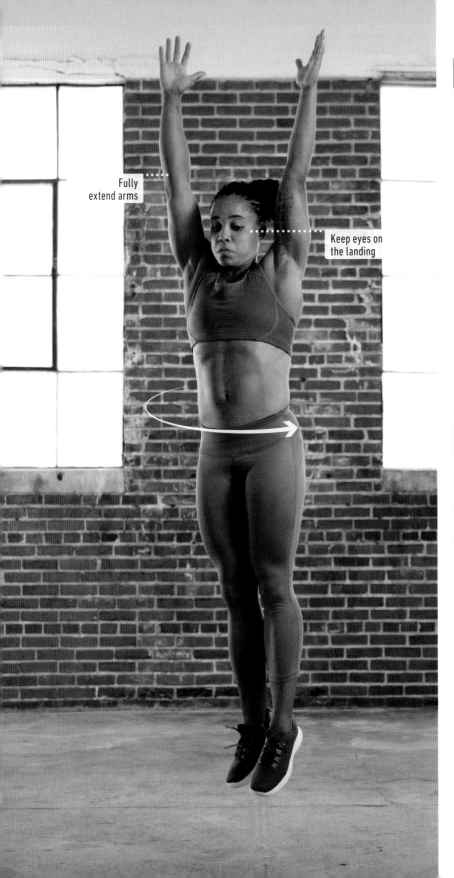

Fully extend arms

Keep eyes on the landing

[3] Forcefully swing your arms up as you explode into a 180-degree jump.

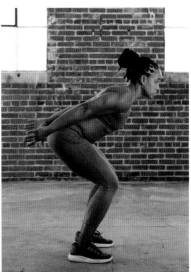

[4] Land softly in a deep squat, and then return to an athletic stance. Repeat the jump in the opposite direction.

MASTERING THE MOVEMENT

GOOD: 1 set of 10
BETTER: 1 set of 20
MASTERED: 1 set of 40

CARIOCA RUN

The Carioca Run strengthens your heart, opens your hips, and improves your mobility to help boost your performance in activities that require dynamic lateral movement.

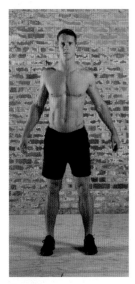

[1] Stand with your feet positioned slightly wider than your hips, with your knees slightly bent and your arms at your sides.

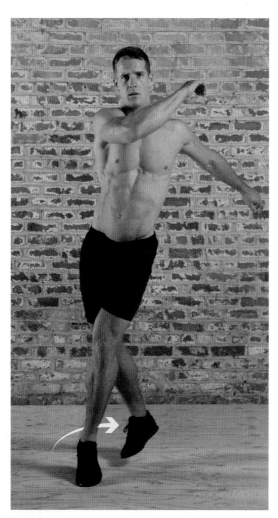

[2] Begin the run to the left by swinging your arms to generate momentum, and simultaneously swinging your right foot behind your body and planting it on the ground.

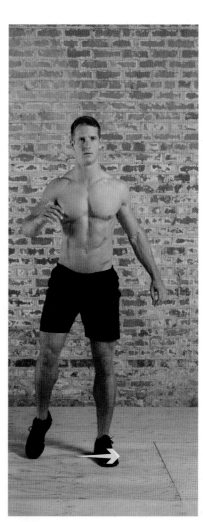

[3] Push off your right foot to step your left foot over.

[4] Push off from your left foot to swing your right foot up and across the front of your body.

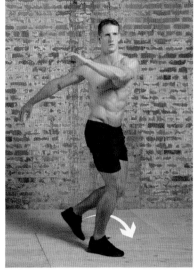

[5] Land on your right foot, and then swing your left foot behind your body.

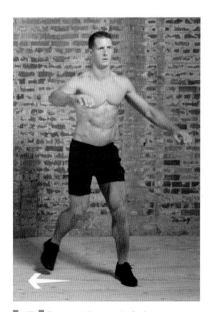

[6] Push off your left foot to step back to the right and reverse the direction of the run. Repeat the movement by rapidly running back and forth in a continuous motion.

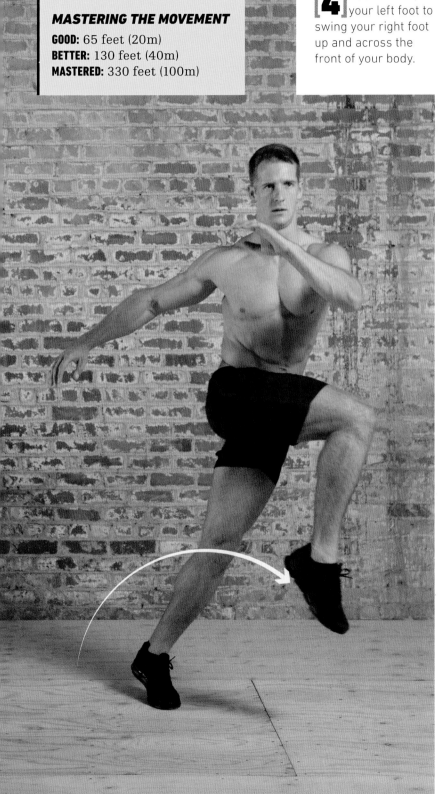

JUMPING LUNGE

The Jumping Lunge, when performed correctly, doesn't require superior strength to execute, but it will boost the explosive power in your lower body by engaging your hips, glutes, and quads.

[1] Begin in a forward lunge position with your weight evenly distributed through your feet. Load your body by extending your arms behind your back.

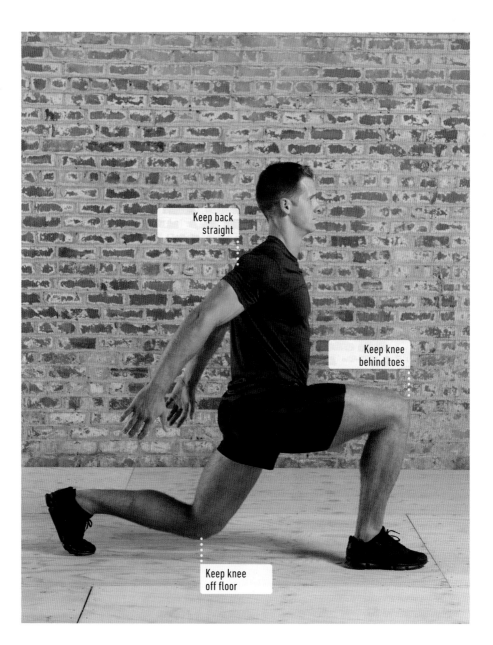

Keep back straight

Keep knee behind toes

Keep knee off floor

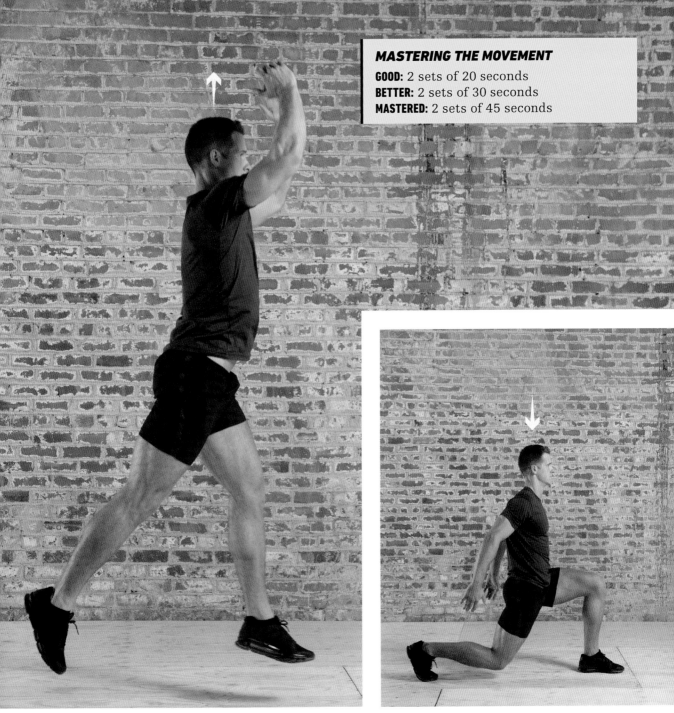

[2] Engage your legs and explode straight up as you swing your arms up over your head and reverse your leg positions at the top of the jump.

[3] Return both arms behind your back as you land softly in the forward lunge position with your leg positions reversed.

BURPEE

Truly a full-body movement, the Burpee will require you to engage nearly every major muscle group in your body to knock out reps of this killer cardio movement.

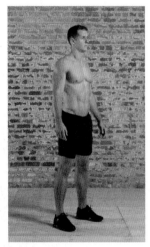

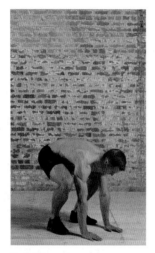

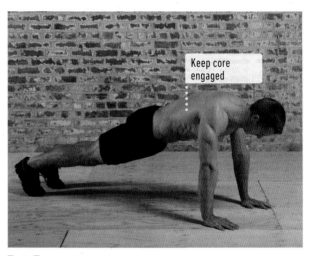

Keep core engaged

[1] Begin in a standing position with your feet positioned shoulder width apart and your arms by your sides.

[2] Lower yourself into a deep squat with your hands placed flat on the floor.

[3] Push through your hands to kick your legs out into a high plank position.

[4] Drop into a low push-up position.

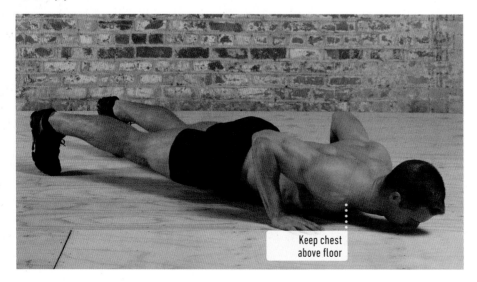

Keep chest above floor

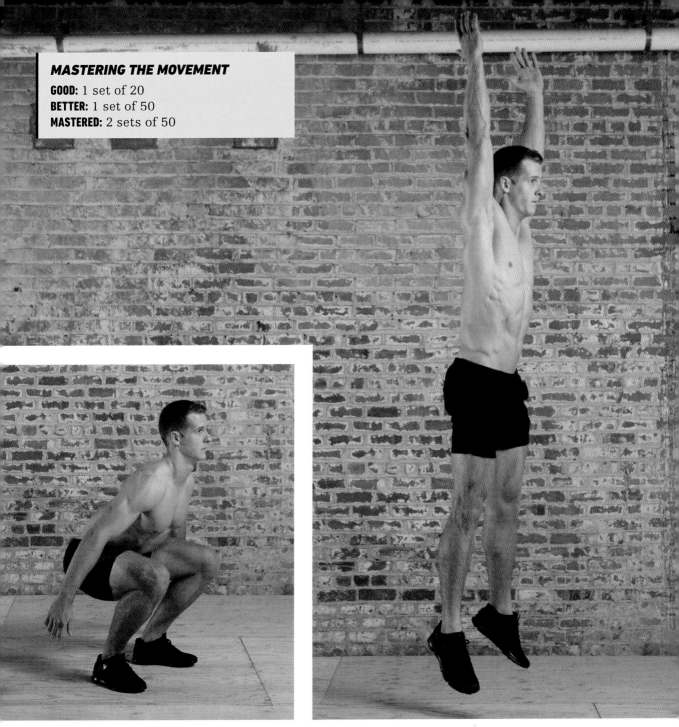

[5] Engage your arms and shoulders to explode up and out of the low push-up position and back into a deep squat, this time with your arms loaded behind you.

[6] Engage your glutes and quads to explode straight up, raising your arms high above your head. Upon landing, drop back down into a high plank position, perform a push-up, and explode back into the starting position.

HURRICANE BURPEE

Even more intense than a Burpee, the Hurricane Burpee will get your heart pounding and your legs and core working even harder by adding in a rotational jumping jack.

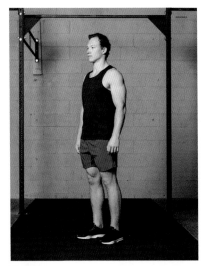

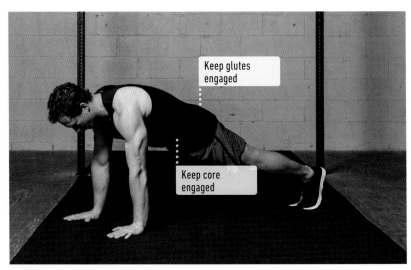

Keep glutes engaged

Keep core engaged

[1] Begin in a standing position with your feet positioned slightly narrower than shoulder width apart, and your arms at your sides.

[2] Drop into a low squat with your hands flat on the ground, and immediately kick your feet back into a high plank position.

[3] Drop into a low push-up position.

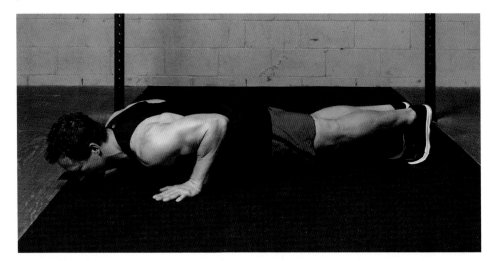

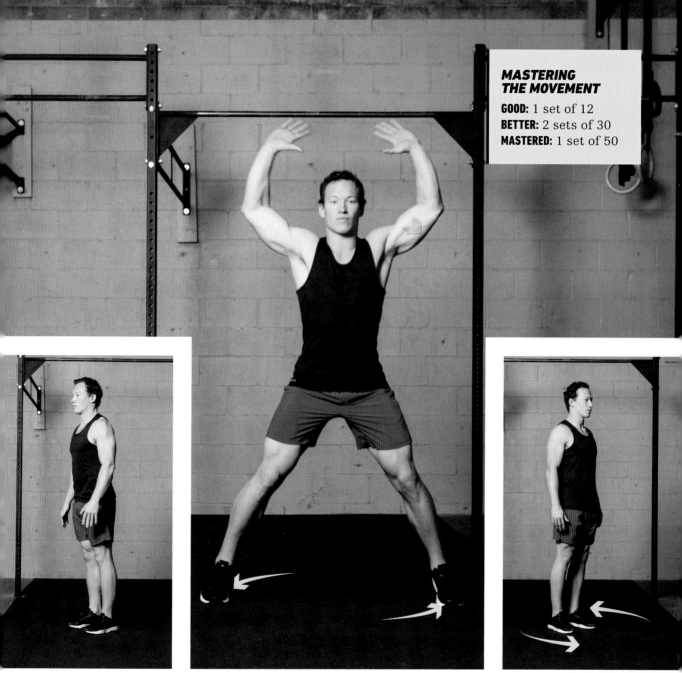

[4] In one explosive motion, push your body up and jump back onto your feet to come into a low squat, and then rise back up into the standing position.

[5] Immediately jump your feet 45 degrees and perform a half jumping jack.

[6] Close the jumping jack with a second 45-degree jump. Repeat the movement as you continue rotating in a circular direction.

SUMO SQUAT JUMP

A basic squat is a tried-and-true calisthenic movement, but the Sumo Squat Jump delivers a new kind of pain—one you're guaranteed to feel in your quads and glutes!

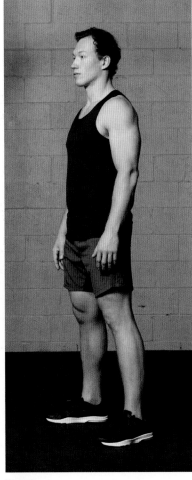

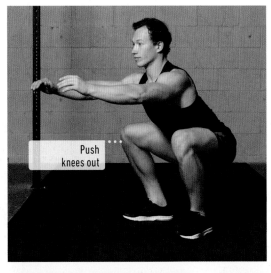

Push knees out

[2] Drop into a low squat position with your back straight, your hips low, and your arms extended straight out in front of you.

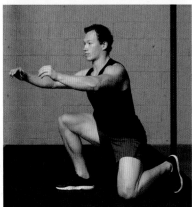

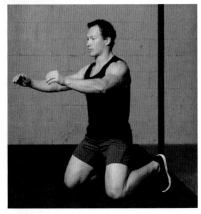

[1] Begin in a standing position with your feet positioned shoulder width apart and your arms at your sides.

[3] Keeping your arms extended in front of you, drop your left knee to the ground.

[4] Next, drop your right knee to the ground.

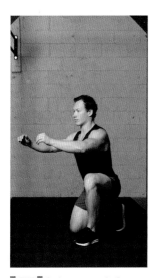

[5] Bring your left knee back up into the squat position.

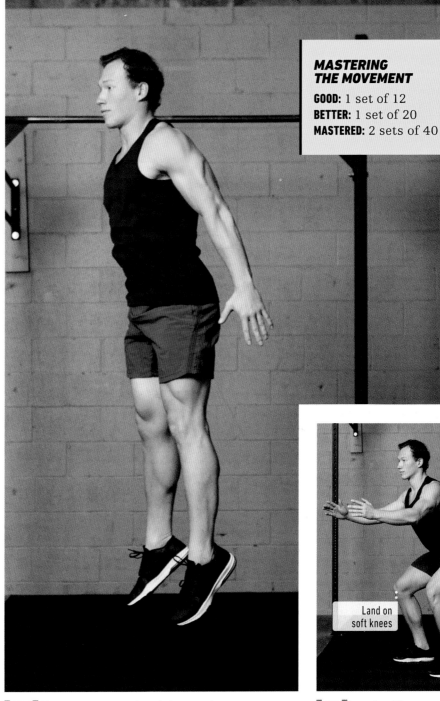

Land on soft knees

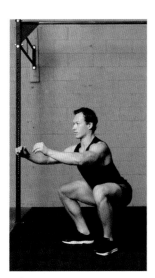

[6] Bring your right knee back up into the squat position.

[7] Engage your quads, glutes, and core, exhale quickly, and explode into the air as high as possible as you extend your arms down to your sides.

[8] Land softly, keeping your knees bent while bringing your arms back up in front of you. Return to the starting position.

BOX JUMP

The Box Jump will improve your body awareness and develop explosive strength in your legs for activities that require jumping movements, such as basketball or parkour.

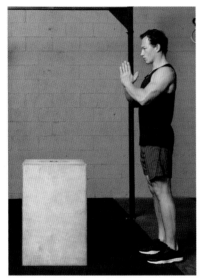

[1] Stand in front of a plyo box with your feet positioned shoulder width apart and your hands pressed together in front of your chest.

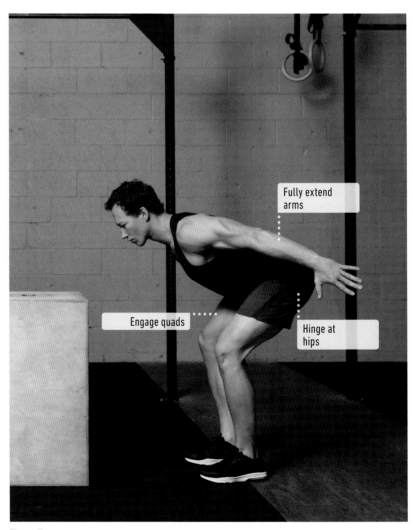

Fully extend arms

Engage quads

Hinge at hips

[2] Drop into a deep squat and extend your arms behind you.

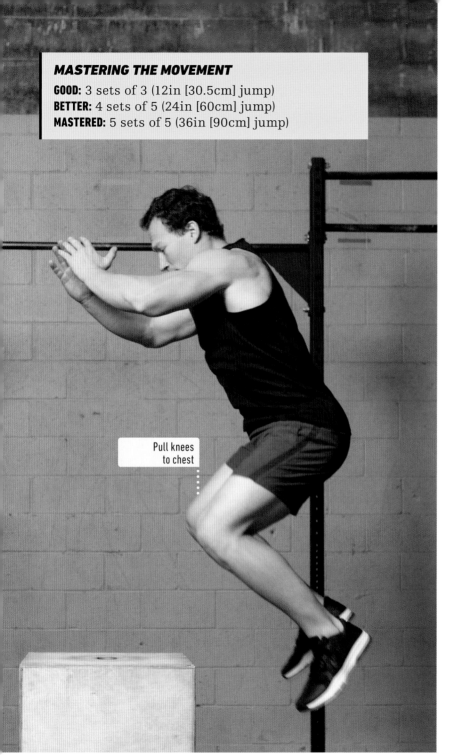

Pull knees to chest

[3] Engage your core and quads and swing your arms up to explode up onto the box.

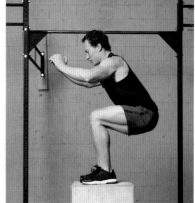

[4] Land softly on the box with your knees bent and positioned directly over your toes.

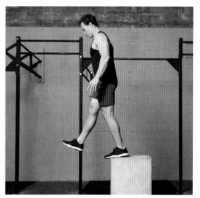

[5] Rise up out of the squat; then step forward and off the box.

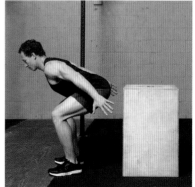

[6] Land softly on bent knees with your hips low and your arms extended behind you.

LATERAL HURDLE JUMP

The Lateral Hurdle Jump will increase your lower body strength, stability, and coordination, and also help reduce the risk of injury by improving your balance and body awareness.

[1] Place a set of parallettes shoulder width apart on the ground. Position yourself next to the parallettes in a low squat position with your feet positioned shoulder width apart and your arms extended behind you.

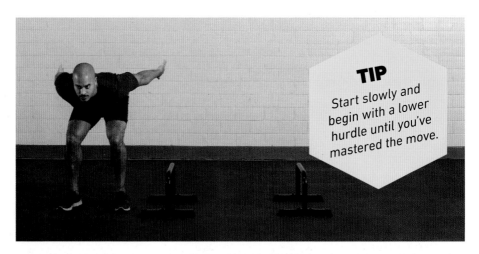

TIP
Start slowly and begin with a lower hurdle until you've mastered the move.

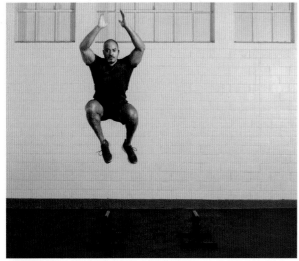

[2] Engage your quads and core, and immediately swing your arms up to explode sideways and over the first hurdle.

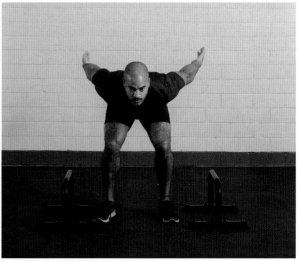

[3] Land softly on both feet with your arms extended back behind you.

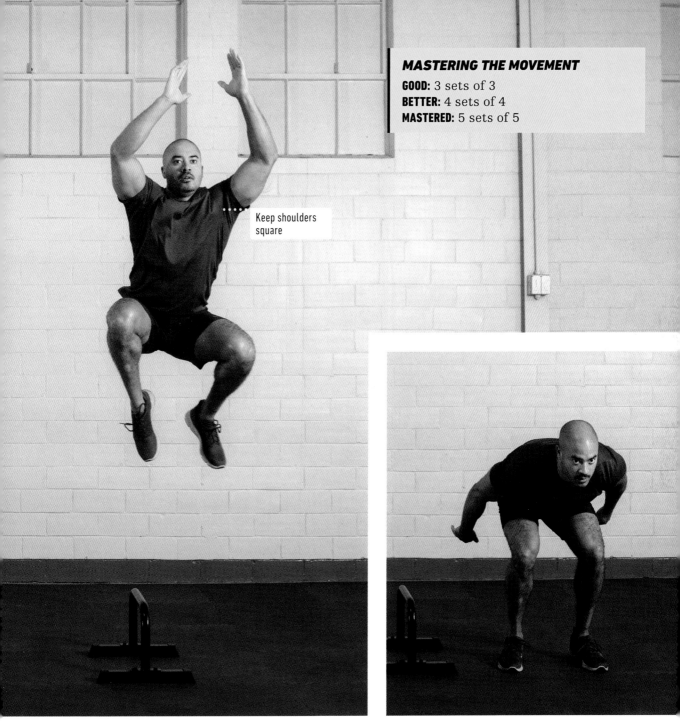

MASTERING THE MOVEMENT

GOOD: 3 sets of 3
BETTER: 4 sets of 4
MASTERED: 5 sets of 5

Keep shoulders square

[4] Once again engage your quads and core to explode into the next jump and over the next hurdle.

[5] Land softly on both feet with your arms extended behind you. Reverse the direction and jump back to the starting position.

BROAD JUMP

The Broad Jump is a complex move that will build explosive strength and requires flexibility and body control. It takes practice and patience to master.

[1] Begin in a standing position with your feet positioned shoulder width apart and your hands in front of your chest; then load your body by dropping into a low squat position with your arms extended behind you.

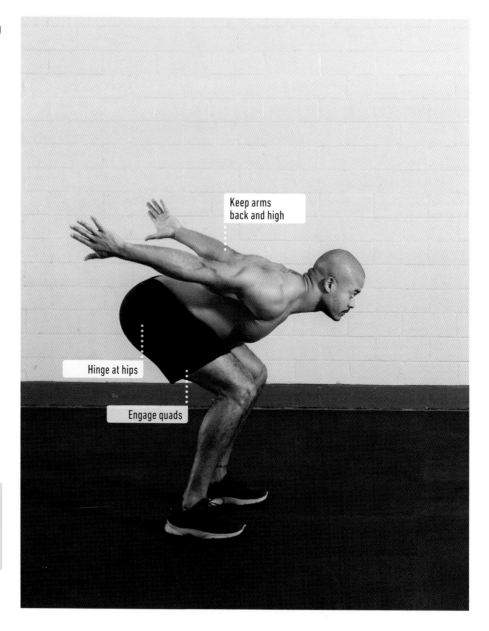

Keep arms back and high

Hinge at hips

Engage quads

TIP
Keep your reps low, go slow, and focus on proper form.

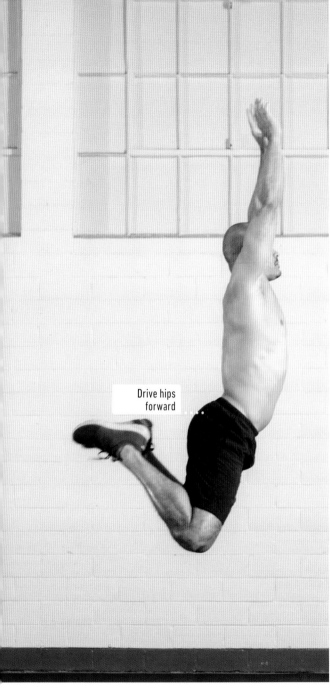

Drive hips forward

MASTERING THE MOVEMENT

GOOD: 2 sets of 5
BETTER: 4 sets of 4 (10% farther)
MASTERED: 4 sets of 3 (20% farther)

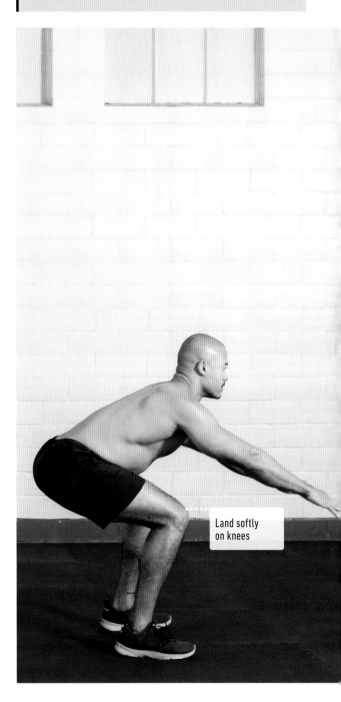

Land softly on knees

[2] Engage your glutes and swing your arms forward and up to explode forward as far as possible.

[3] Bring your arms back down in front of you as you land softly on bent knees, and drop back into a low squat position.

BOX-TO-BROAD JUMP

The Box-to-Broad Jump is a dynamic plyometric exercise that combines the explosive power of box jumps and broad jumps. Your quads will be screaming after a few of these!

[1] Begin by standing in front of a plyo box with your feet positioned shoulder width apart and your hands pressed together in front of your chest; then load your body by dropping into a low squat with your arms extended behind you.

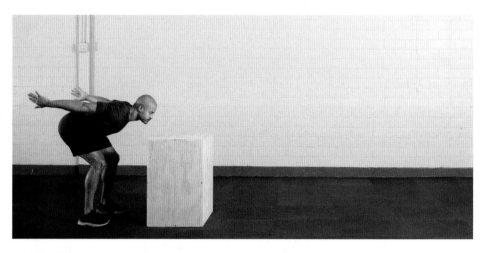

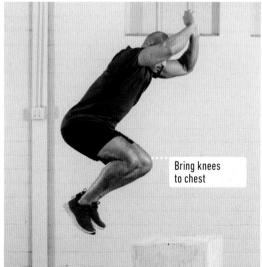

Bring knees to chest

[2] Engage your core and quads and forcefully swing your arms up as you explode up and onto the box.

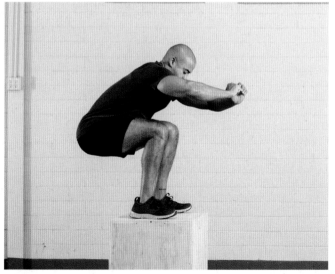

[3] Land softly on the box on flat feet with your knees positioned directly behind your toes.

[4] Rise up out of the squat; then step forward and off the box.

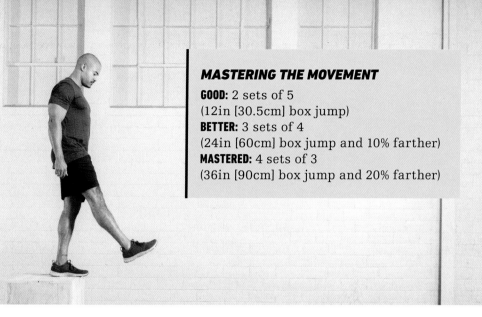

MASTERING THE MOVEMENT

GOOD: 2 sets of 5
(12in [30.5cm] box jump)
BETTER: 3 sets of 4
(24in [60cm] box jump and 10% farther)
MASTERED: 4 sets of 3
(36in [90cm] box jump and 20% farther)

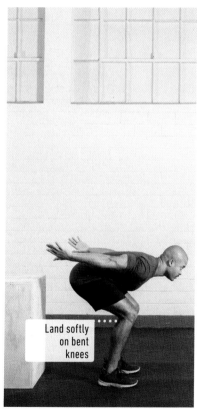

Land softly on bent knees

[5] Land softly into a deep squat position with your knees bent and your arms extended behind you.

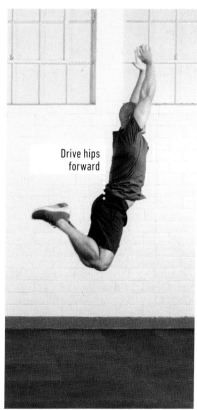

Drive hips forward

[6] Engage your core and quads, and swing your arms up, as you explode forward as far as possible.

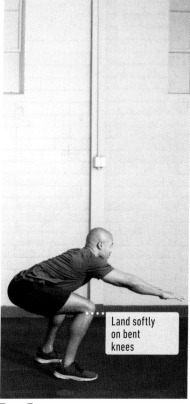

Land softly on bent knees

[7] Land softly on flat feet and bent knees as you bring your arms back down in front of you.

DOUBLE BROAD JUMP

The Double Broad Jump is a serious test of athleticism that will challenge your entire lower body. Perfect your technique before propelling yourself through multiple jumps.

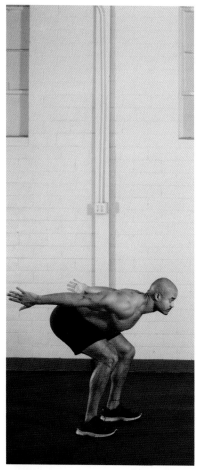 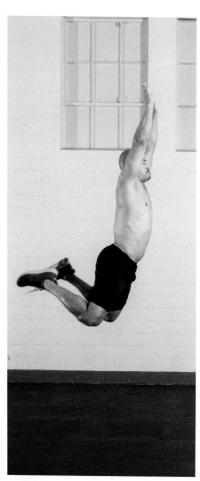 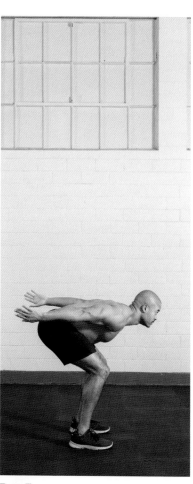

[1] Begin in a standing position with your feet positioned shoulder width apart and your hands pressed together in front of your chest; then load your body by dropping into a low squat position with your arms extended behind you.

[2] Engage your quads and core and swing your arms up to explode forward as far as possible.

[3] Land softly on flat feet as you bring your arms back down behind you.

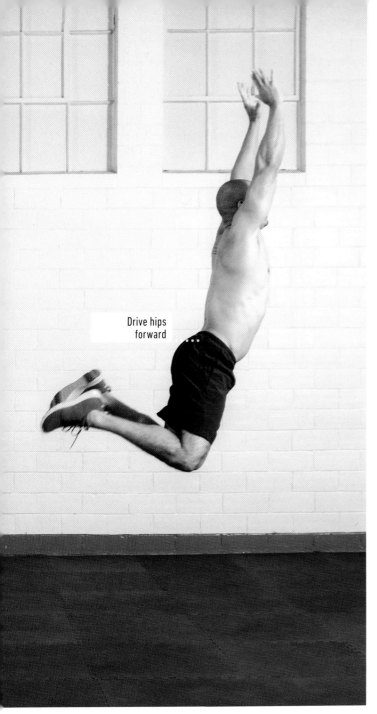

Drive hips forward

MASTERING THE MOVEMENT
GOOD: 2 sets of 5
BETTER: 3 sets of 4 (10% farther)
MASTERED: 4 sets of 3 (20% farther)

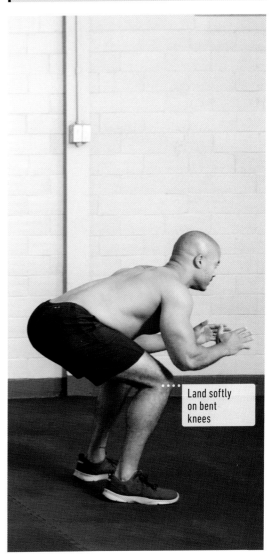

Land softly on bent knees

[4] Immediately engage your quads and core and swing your arms up to explode forward as far as possible.

[5] Land softly on flat feet and bent knees as you bring your arms back down in front of you. Return to a standing position and repeat the movement.

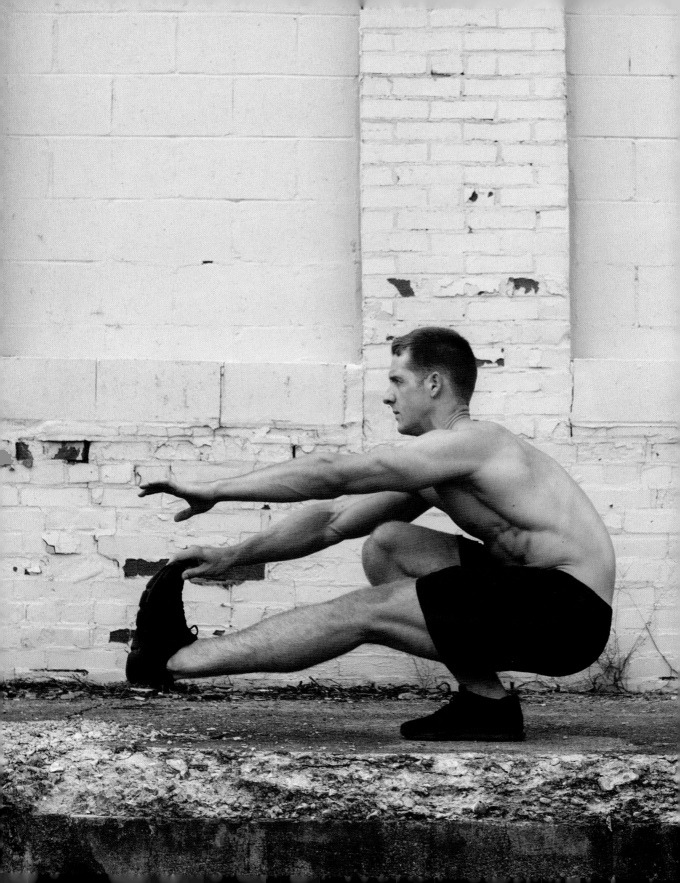

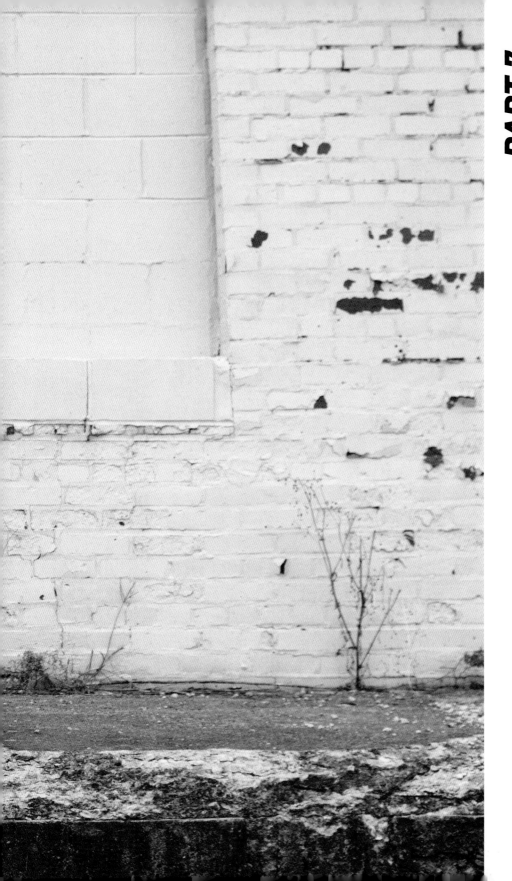

LUNGE

The Lunge builds strength in the entire lower body, increases mobility in the hamstrings and hip flexors, and can help improve balance and coordination.

[1] Begin in a standing position with your feet positioned shoulder width apart and your arms at your sides.

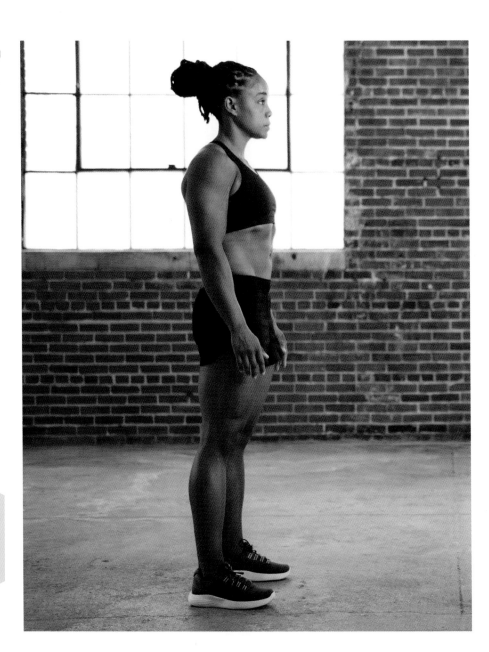

TIP
When starting out, first take a step forward then drop into the lunge.

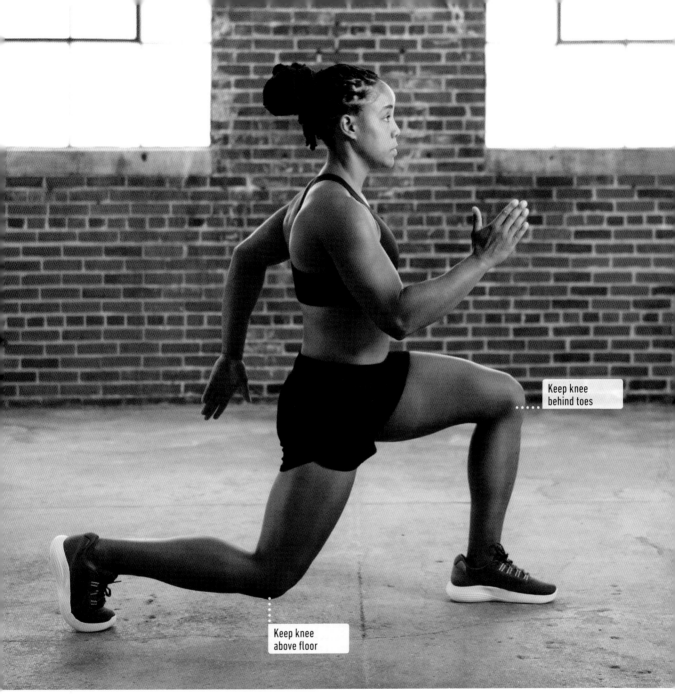

Keep knee
behind toes

Keep knee
above floor

[2] Drop into a lunge by pushing from your right foot and stepping your left foot forward while simultaneously swinging your right arm up and your left arm back. Return to the starting position by pushing through your left heel; then reverse your arm and leg positions and repeat on the opposite side.

MASTERING THE MOVEMENT

GOOD: 3 alternating sets of 10
BETTER: 2 alternating sets of 25
MASTERED: 1 alternating set of 50

SIDE LUNGE

The Side Lunge will build strength and dynamic flexibility in your legs and improve your hip stability. It's excellent for athletes who need power in lateral outstretched positions.

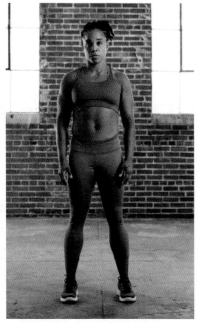

[1] Begin in a standing position with your feet positioned slightly wider than shoulder width apart and your arms at your sides.

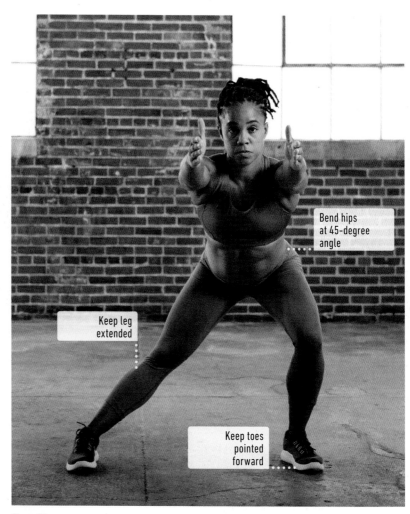

Bend hips at 45-degree angle

Keep leg extended

Keep toes pointed forward

[2] In a controlled fashion, swing your arms up in front you and step to your left as far as possible while fully extending your right leg.

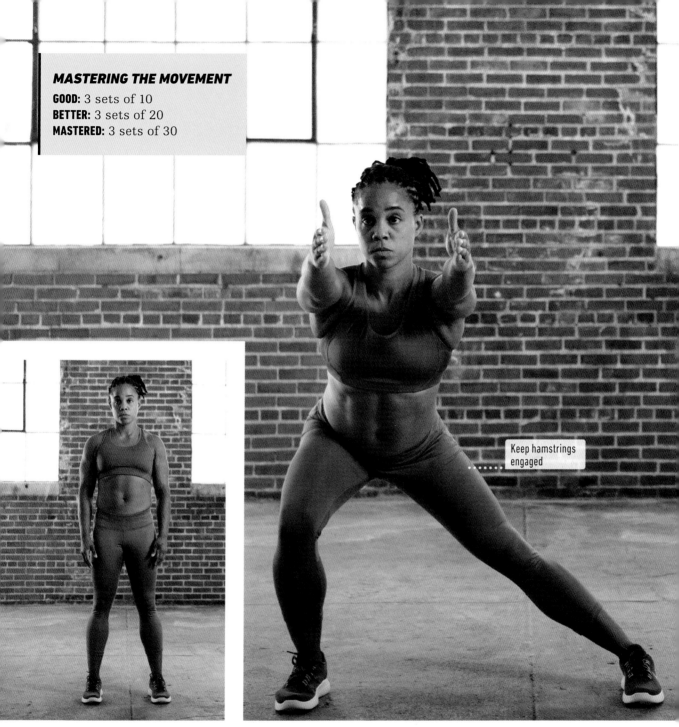

Keep hamstrings engaged

[3] Push off from your left foot to return to the starting position.

[4] In a controlled fashion, swing your arms up in front you and step to your right as far as possible while fully extending your left leg; then push from your right foot to return to the starting position.

AIR SQUAT

The Air Squat is a simple movement, but it builds excellent lower body strength. It won't take long before you begin to feel some serious burn in your hamstrings and quads!

[1] Begin in a standing position with your feet positioned shoulder width apart. Roll your shoulders back and down, and extend your arms straight out in front of you with your thumbs pointing up.

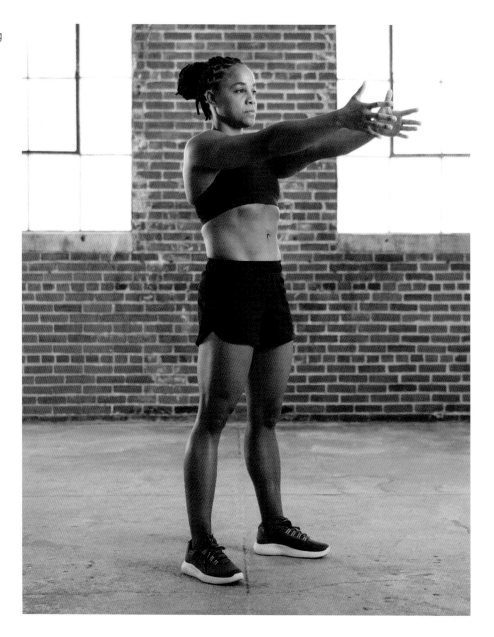

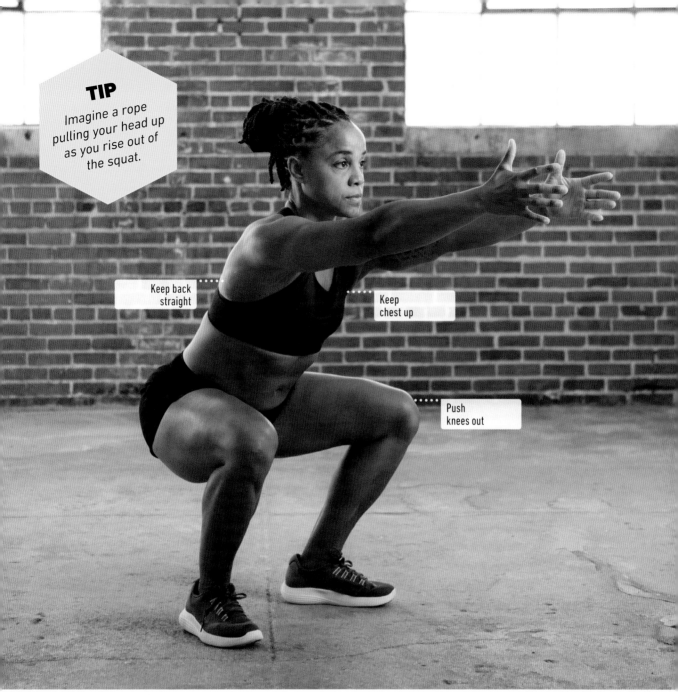

TIP
Imagine a rope pulling your head up as you rise out of the squat.

Keep back straight

Keep chest up

Push knees out

[2] Drop straight down into a low squat until your thighs are parallel to the ground; then rise back up into the starting position.

MASTERING THE MOVEMENT

GOOD: 3 sets of 10
BETTER: 2 sets of 25
MASTERED: 1 set of 50

GLUTE BRIDGE AND MARCH

The Glute Bridge and March is a phenomenal lower-body exercise that will activate your core and develop powerful strength in your glutes, hips, and hamstrings.

[1] Lie on your back with your your feet flat on the ground, your knees bent, and your arms extended away from your body. Push your lower back into the ground to activate your core.

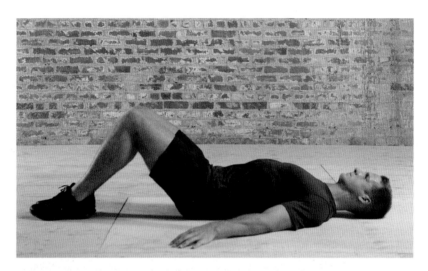

[2] Contract your hamstrings and glutes and push through your heels to elevate your hips off the ground.

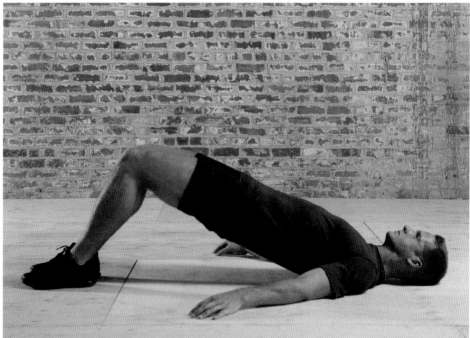

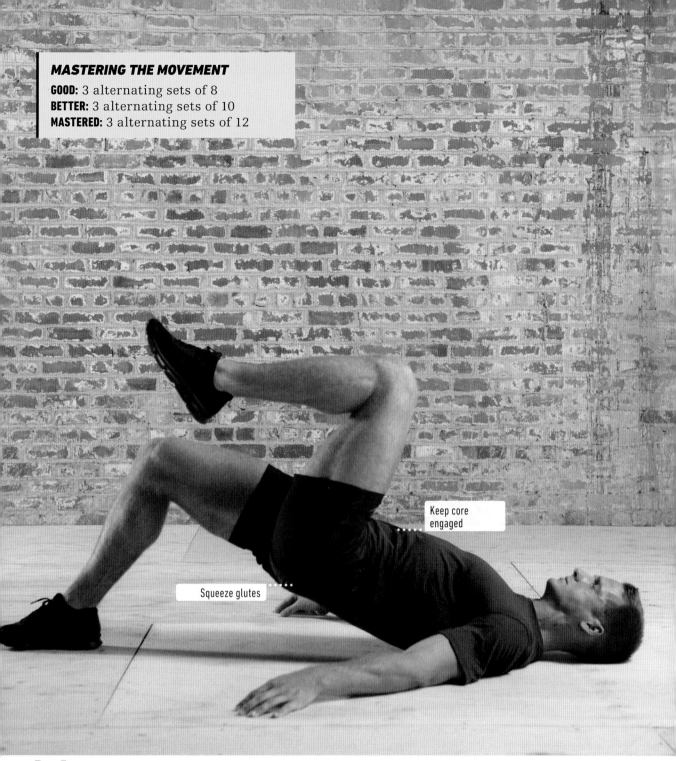

MASTERING THE MOVEMENT
GOOD: 3 alternating sets of 8
BETTER: 3 alternating sets of 10
MASTERED: 3 alternating sets of 12

Keep core engaged

Squeeze glutes

[3] At the top of the bridge, alternate raising each leg toward your chest in a marching motion.

WALL SIT

Static, or *isometric*, exercises build strength by maintaining muscular contraction against resistance. The Wall Sit is a fantastic isometric exercise for building strength in your glutes and quads.

[1] Stand with your back flat against a wall and your feet shoulder width apart and positioned approximately 20 inches (.50m) away from the wall. Place your hands on your thighs.

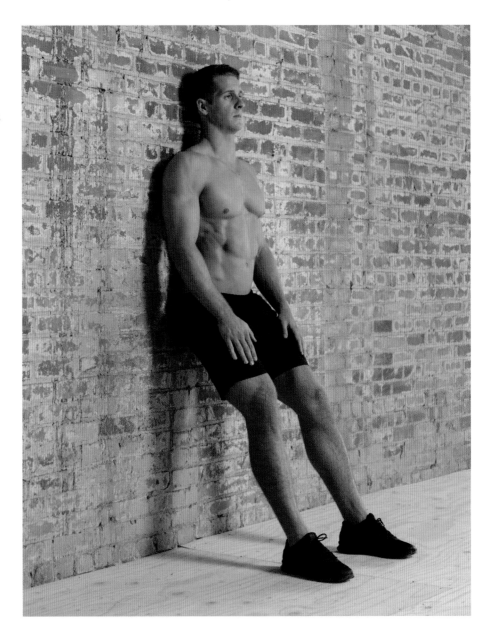

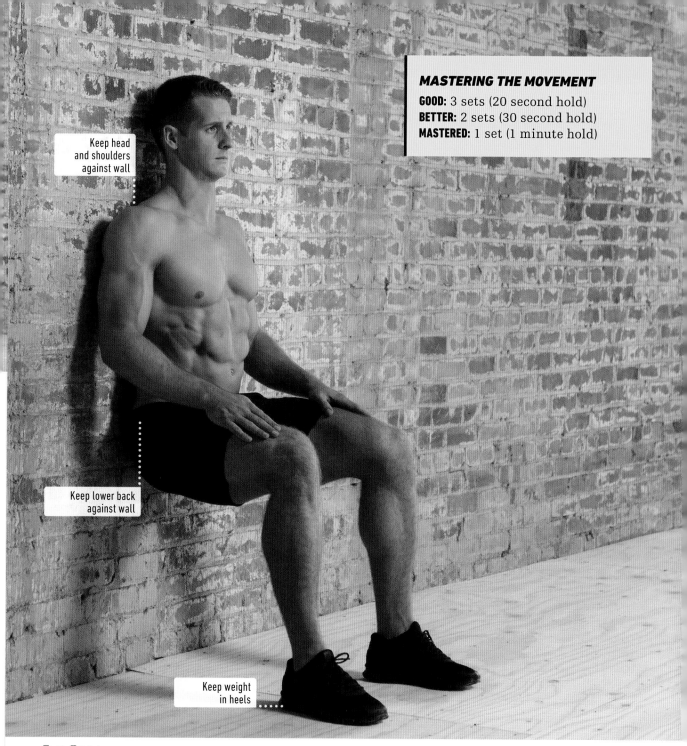

Keep head
and shoulders
against wall

MASTERING THE MOVEMENT
GOOD: 3 sets (20 second hold)
BETTER: 2 sets (30 second hold)
MASTERED: 1 set (1 minute hold)

Keep lower back
against wall

Keep weight
in heels

[2] Slide your back down the wall until your hips
and knees are bent at a 90-degree angle and
your thighs are parallel to the ground. Hold, and then
push your body back up into the starting position.

EXPLOSIVE KNEE JUMP

The Explosive Knee Jump requires your central nervous system to fire on all cylinders. Once you've mastered it, you'll be able to jump higher, leap farther, sprint faster, and kick harder.

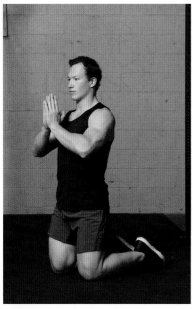

[1] Begin in a kneeling position, with your legs positioned slightly wider than your hips, your back straight, and your hands pressed together in front of your chest.

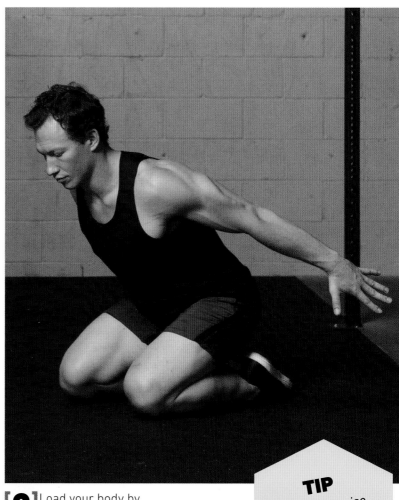

[2] Load your body by extending your arms behind you, lowering your glutes toward your legs, and lowering your chest toward the ground.

TIP
Use an exercise mat to help cushion your knees.

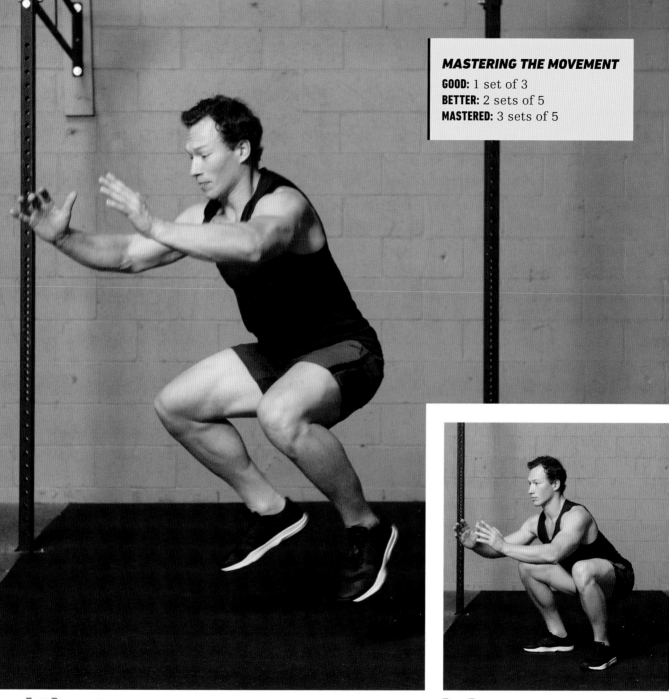

[3] In one fluid motion, forcefully swing your arms up and explode from your knees.

[4] Land softly on your feet in a low squat position; then return to the starting position by lowering your knees back to ground, one at a time.

HAMSTRING CURL

This movement will absolutely torch your hamstrings! Using a towel will help isolate the hamstrings and speed up the size and strength progression.

[1] Place a folded towel on a slick surface. Lie on your back with your arms extended to your sides. Place your heels on the towel and lift your hips up into a bridge position.

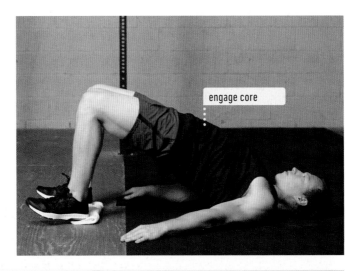

engage core

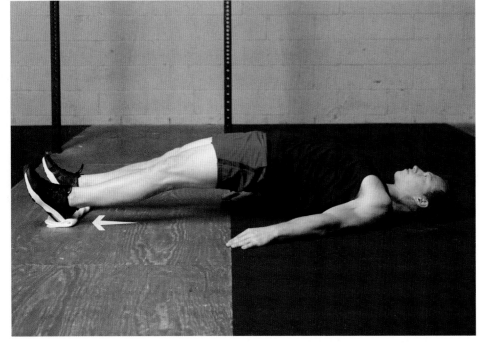

[2] Engage your glutes and abs, and slide your feet out until your legs are extended, but your hips are still elevated off the ground.

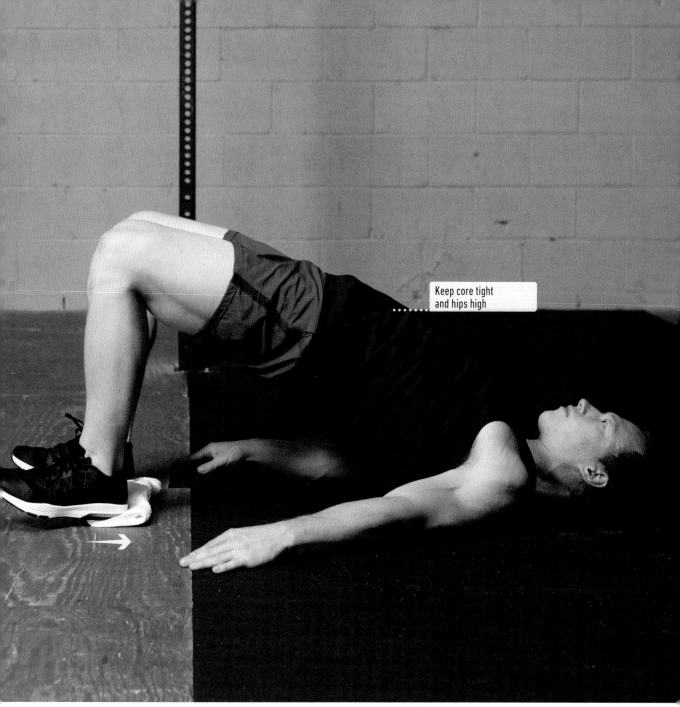

Keep core tight
and hips high

[3] Flex at your knees and hips to slide your feet back toward your glutes until they're directly beneath your knees. Repeat in a back-and-forth sliding motion.

MASTERING THE MOVEMENT

GOOD: 2 sets of 6
BETTER: 3 sets of 6
MASTERED: 4 sets of 6

NORDIC HAMSTRING CURL

The Nordic Hamstring Curl strengthens weakened posterior muscles, helps increase your speed and agility, and can help prevent debilitating hamstring injuries.

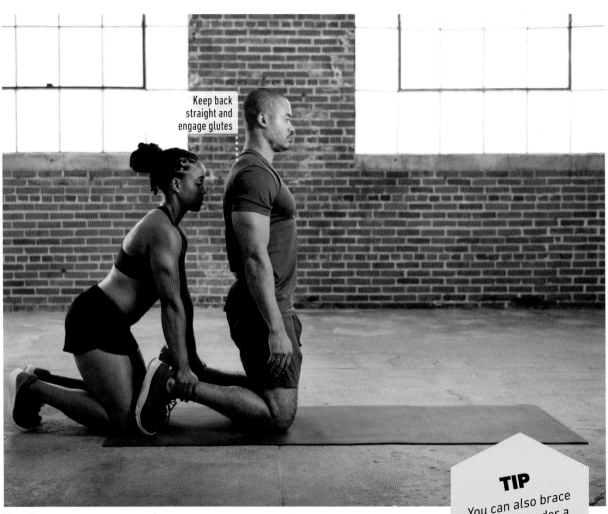

Keep back straight and engage glutes

TIP
You can also brace your feet under a bench or low bar.

[1] Begin in a kneeling position with your arms at your sides. Have a partner brace your ankles to secure your feet.

[2] Take a deep breath and lower yourself to the ground as slowly as possible while keeping your body straight and tight, and keeping your hamstrings and core engaged during the descent.

MASTERING THE MOVEMENT

GOOD: 2 sets of 3
BETTER: 3 sets of 5
MASTERED: 4 sets of 5

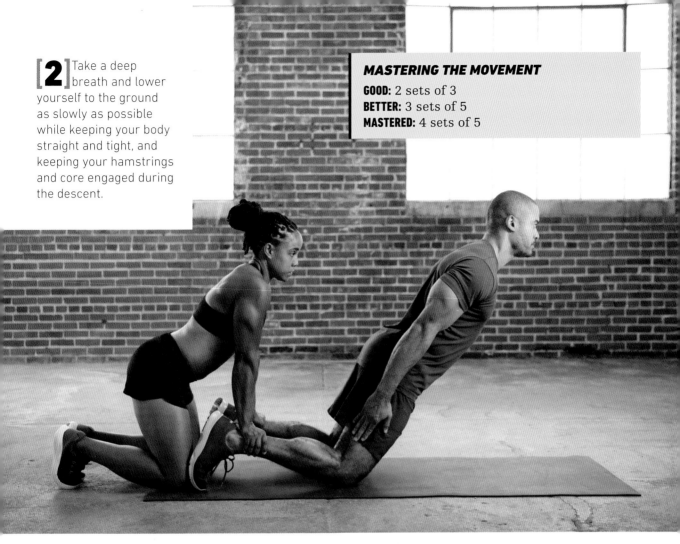

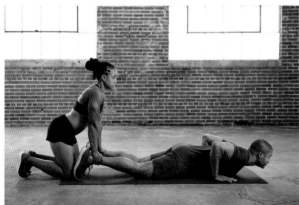

[3] Land softly on your hands.

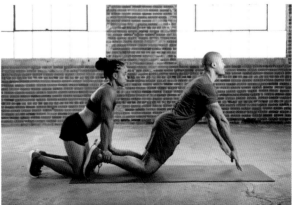

[4] Engage your shoulders and arms to explosively push yourself back up into the starting position.

SHRIMP SQUAT

The Shrimp Squat targets the quads and glutes. Flexing the nonsquatting leg toward the glute further enhances the movement to help develop more lower body mobility and strength.

[1] Begin in a standing position with your feet positioned shoulder width apart. Bend at your knee to bring one foot up behind your body, grasping your ankle to pull your foot close to your glute. Extend the opposite arm directly in front of you for balance.

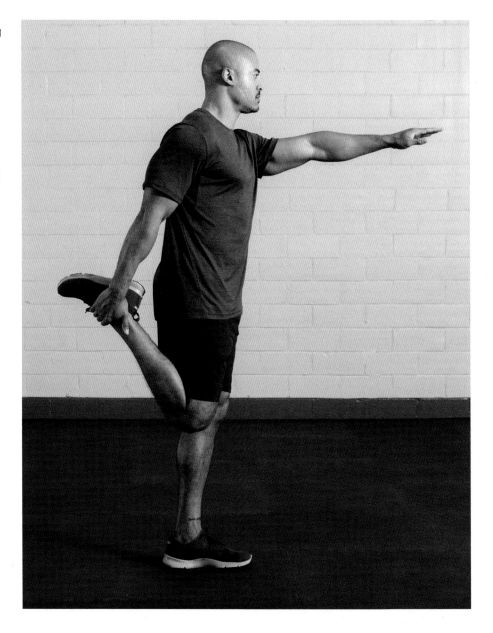

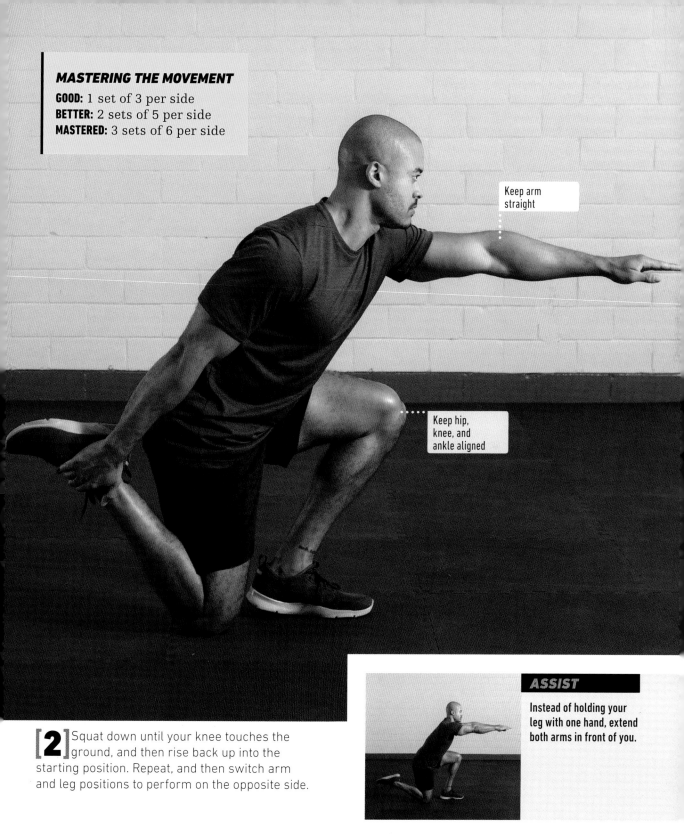

MASTERING THE MOVEMENT
GOOD: 1 set of 3 per side
BETTER: 2 sets of 5 per side
MASTERED: 3 sets of 6 per side

Keep arm
straight

Keep hip,
knee, and
ankle aligned

ASSIST

Instead of holding your
leg with one hand, extend
both arms in front of you.

[2] Squat down until your knee touches the
ground, and then rise back up into the
starting position. Repeat, and then switch arm
and leg positions to perform on the opposite side.

PISTOL SQUAT

The Pistol Squat is a serious calisthenics move that requires a complex mix of strength, flexibility, and motor control to master. There's no turning back now —so let's do this!

[1] Begin in a standing position with your feet positioned shoulder width apart and your arms at your sides. Extend your arms straight in front of you with your palms facing the ground, and slowly raise one leg out in front of you.

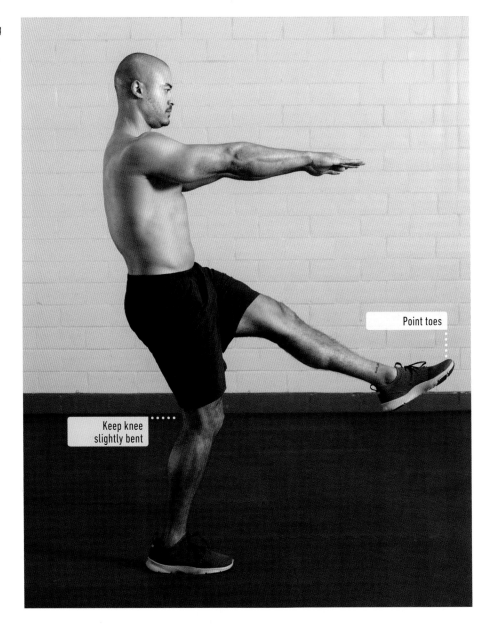

Point toes

Keep knee slightly bent

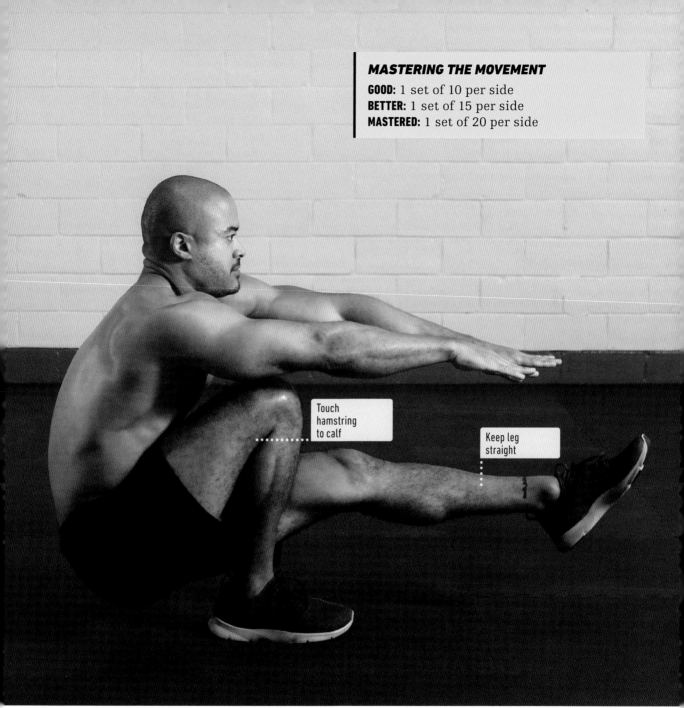

MASTERING THE MOVEMENT

GOOD: 1 set of 10 per side
BETTER: 1 set of 15 per side
MASTERED: 1 set of 20 per side

Touch
hamstring
to calf

Keep leg
straight

[2] Slowly descend into a low squat position,
keeping your front leg fully extended.
In a controlled fashion, push through your
heel to rise back up into the starting position.
Repeat, and then reverse leg positions
to perform on the opposite side.

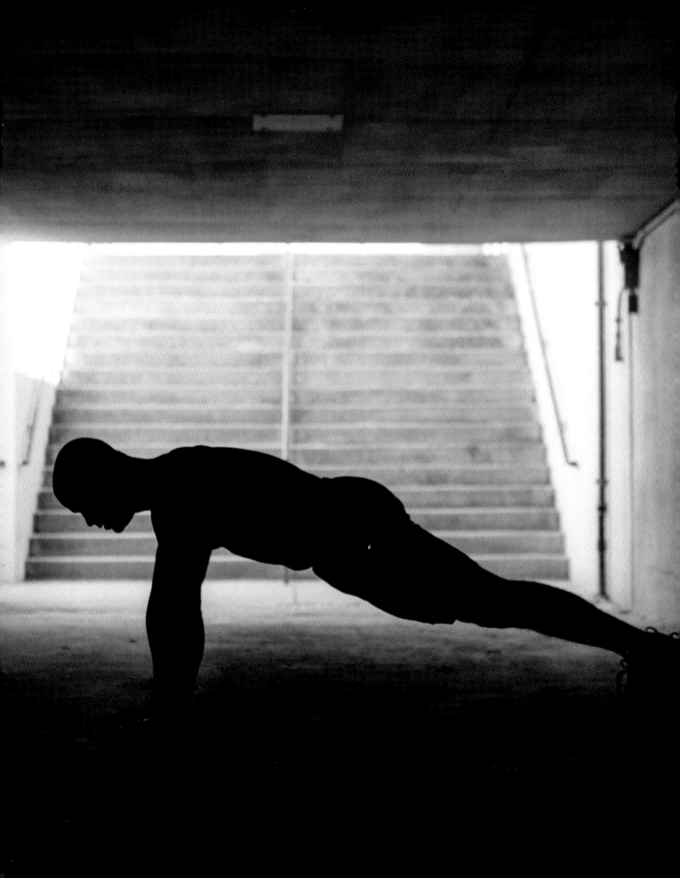

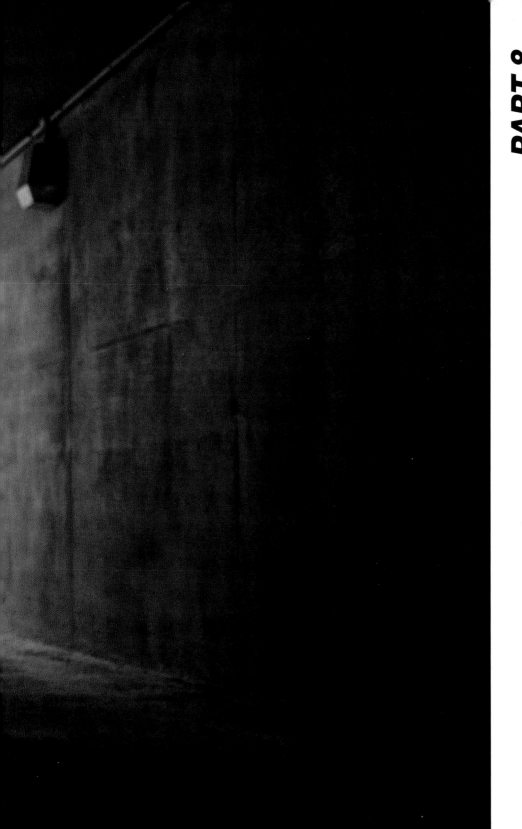

TURKISH GET-UP

The Turkish Get-Up is a classic move that requires your core to constantly be firing as you bend, twist, and lunge to strengthen your torso and increase your body stability.

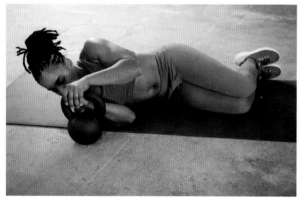

[1] Place a kettlebell next to you on the ground, positioned chest high on your right side. Lie on your right side with your knees bent at 90-degree angles. Grasp the kettlebell with both hands using opposing grips.

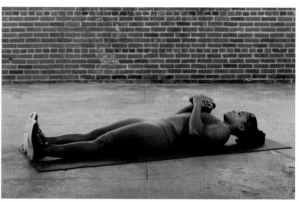

[2] Extend your legs and roll onto your back using both hands to pull the kettlebell up and onto your chest.

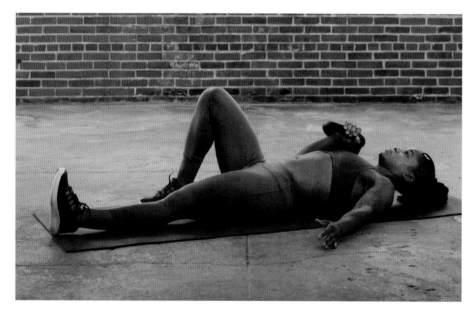

[3] Extend your left arm to your side and slide your right foot up until your knee is bent and your foot is flat on the ground.

[4] Press the kettlebell straight overhead.

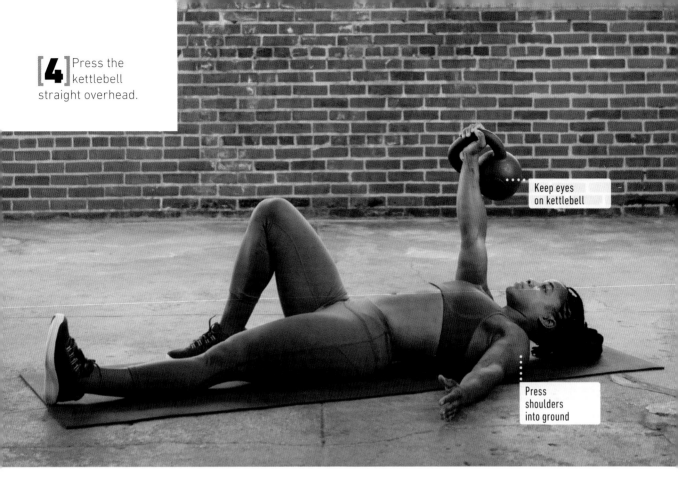

Keep eyes on kettlebell

Press shoulders into ground

[5] Slide your left elbow in toward your body, and then rise up onto your left forearm as you press the kettlebell further skyward.

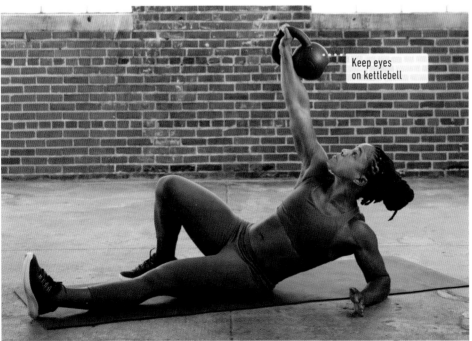

Keep eyes on kettlebell

continues ❯

[6] Press the kettlebell further skyward as you push through your left forearm and rise up until your left arm is fully extended.

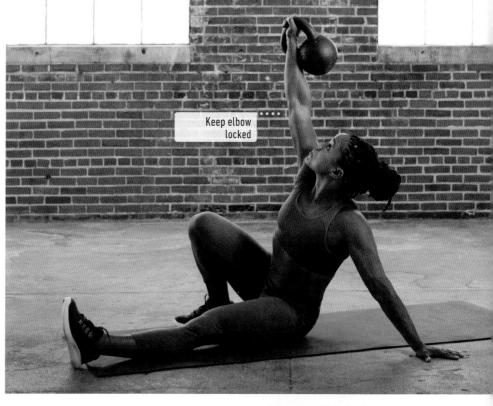

Keep elbow locked

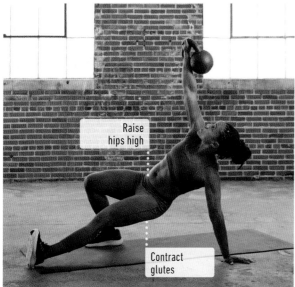

Raise hips high

Contract glutes

[7] Contract your glutes and elevate your hips until your left leg is fully extended and supported on your left heel.

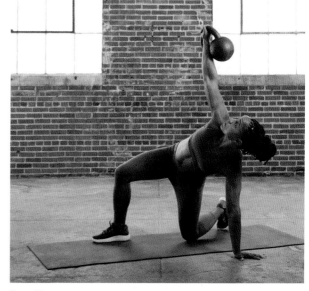

[8] Slide your left leg under and behind you until you're resting on your left knee, keeping the kettlebell steady and your left hand flat on the ground.

Keep eyes on kettlebell

Keep back straight

Keep knee behind toes

MASTERING THE MOVEMENT
GOOD: 1 set of 5 per side
BETTER: 2 sets of 10 per side
MASTERED: 3 sets of 12 per side

[9] Push through your left hand to rise up and press the kettlebell further skyward.

[10] Press the kettlebell up to its highest point by slowly pushing from your left foot, and pushing through your right leg to rise up until your body is erect and you're standing flat on both feet. Reverse the motion to complete the rep.

DOUBLE-LEG MOUNTAIN CLIMBER

The Double-Leg Mountain Climber is an excellent multijoint movement that will take your hips and legs through a big range of motion and get your heart pumping.

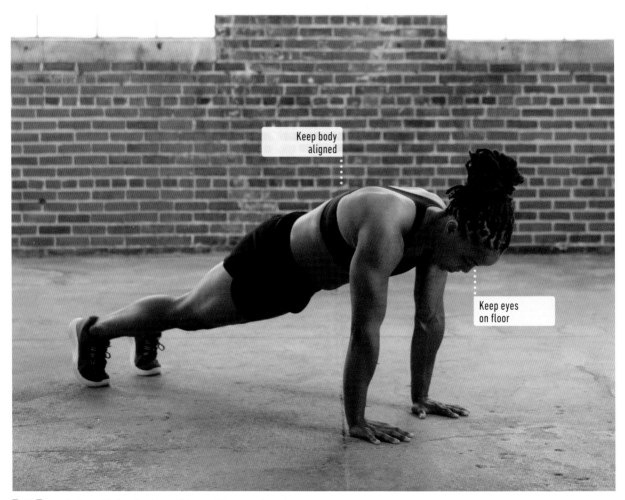

Keep body aligned

Keep eyes on floor

[1] Begin in a high plank position with your hands directly below your shoulders and your feet positioned shoulder width apart. Keep your core engaged, your body straight, and your shoulders pushed down and away from your ears.

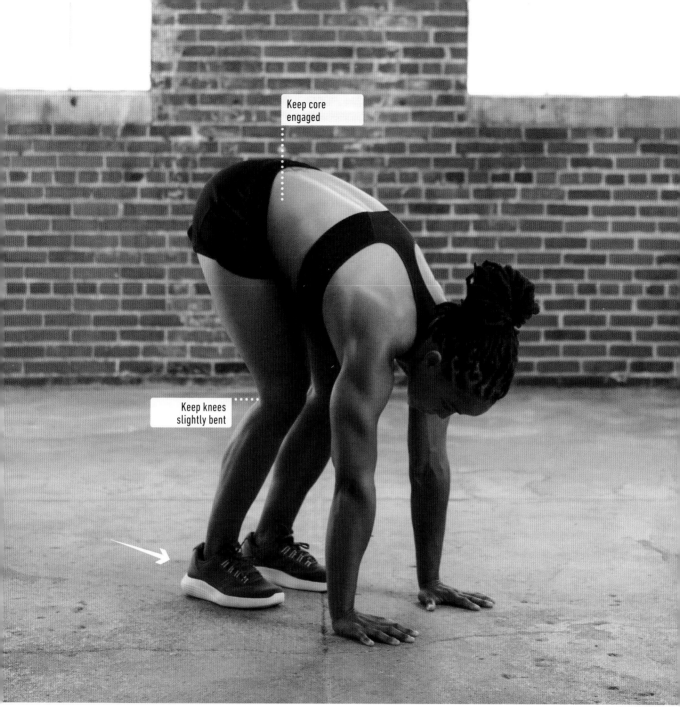

Keep core engaged

Keep knees slightly bent

[2] Squeeze your glutes and thrust your hips skyward as you jump both feet forward toward your hands and then jump them back to the starting position. Repeat the movement in a rapid back-and-forth motion.

MASTERING THE MOVEMENT

GOOD: 1 set of 10
BETTER: 2 sets of 15
MASTERED: 1 set of 30

NINJA PUSH-UP

The Ninja Push-Up requires excellent hip mobility and good upper-body strength to master, but it will develop superior strength in your pecs, triceps, and lower abdominals.

[1] Begin in a high plank position with your hands positioned directly below your shoulders and your feet positioned slightly narrower than shoulder width apart. Push your shoulders down and away from your ears.

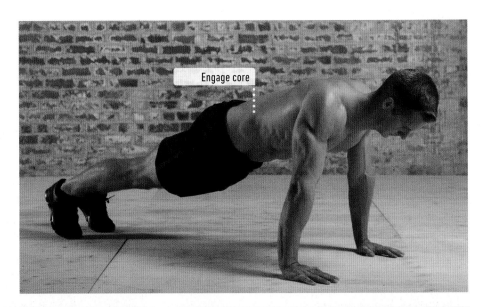

Engage core

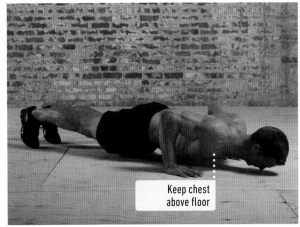

Keep chest above floor

[2] Drop into a low push-up position.

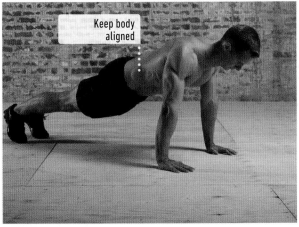

Keep body aligned

[3] Engage your arms and shoulders to push yourself back up into the high plank position.

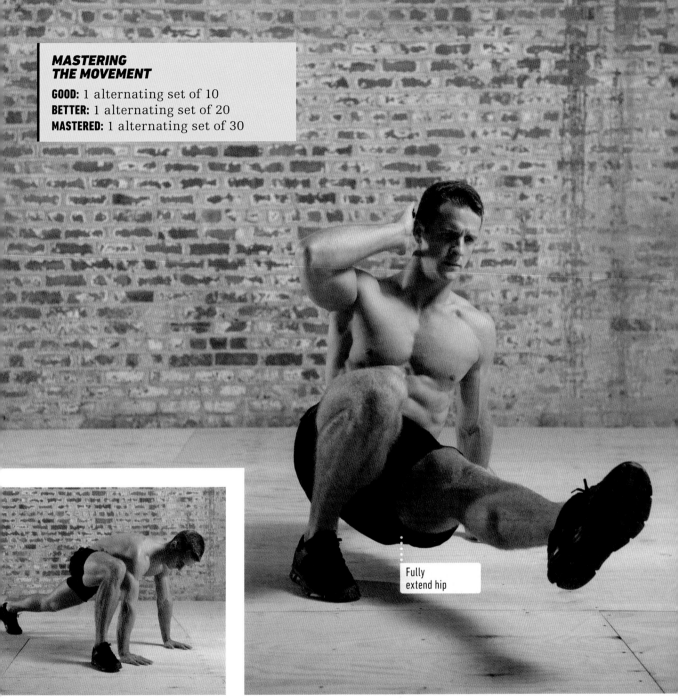

Fully extend hip

[4] Step your right foot forward to align with your right hand.

[5] In one fluid motion, swing your left leg under your body and forward until it's fully extended in front of you, rock your torso back, and bring your right hand up behind your head. Reverse the movement until you're back in a high plank position, and then repeat the movement on the opposite side.

DRAGON WALK

The Dragon Walk is a unilateral staggered movement and is one of the most difficult push-up variations to execute. It will require you to engage nearly every major muscle group in your body.

[1] Begin in a high plank position with your hands directly below your shoulders and your feet positioned slightly narrower than shoulder width apart. Push your shoulders down and away from your ears.

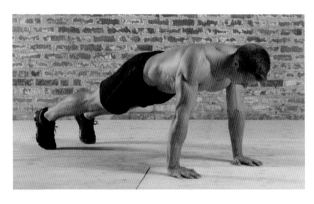

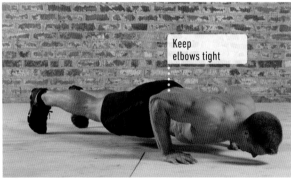

Keep elbows tight

[2] Drop into a low push-up position.

[3] Begin walking forward by pushing yourself up and out of the low push-up position while simultaneously extending your left arm straight in front of you and extending your right leg straight behind you.

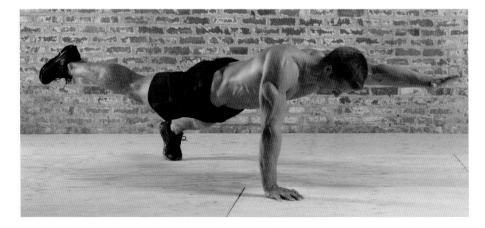

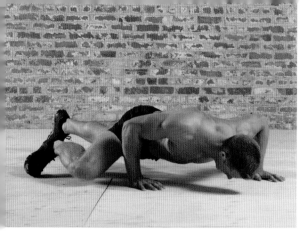

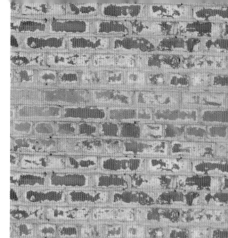

[4] Drop back into a low staggered push-up position, bringing your right knee forward to your elbow as you anchor the toes of your right foot in the ground.

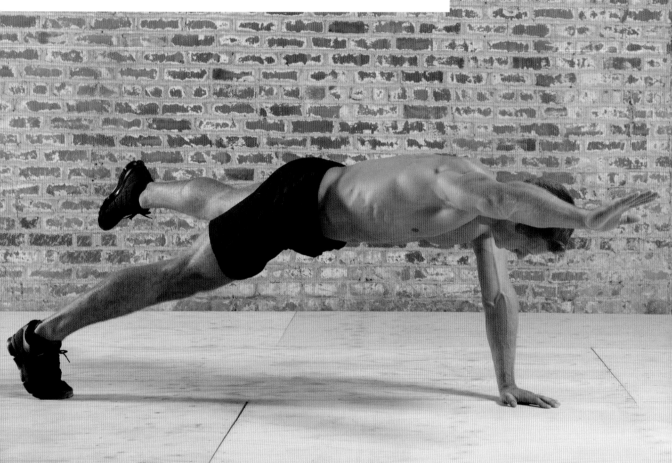

[5] Walk your body forward by pushing from your right foot to come back up into a high plank position while extending your right arm straight in front of you and extending your left leg straight behind you. Alternate your arm and leg positions as you continue to walk forward.

MASTERING THE MOVEMENT

GOOD: 1 set of 10
BETTER: 1 set of 20
MASTERED: 1 set of 30

WINDSHIELD WIPER

The Windshield Wiper requires a strong back as well as serious core stability and strength. It takes time and patience to master, but seeing it executed properly is a site to behold.

[1] Begin in a dead-hang position with your hands placed on the bar in an overhand grip position and positioned slightly wider than shoulder width apart.

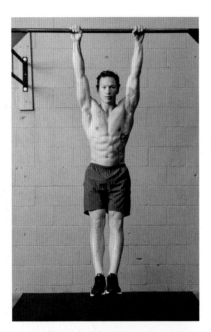

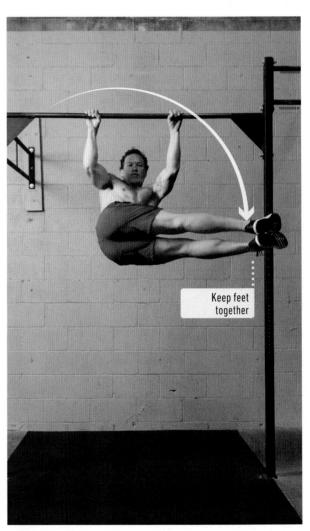

Keep feet together

[2] Engage your lats and contract your upper back to pull your body up until your arms are at 90-degree angles; then engage your core to swing your extended legs up until they're vertical.

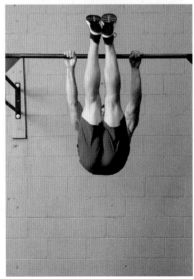

[3] In a controlled fashion, rotate your hips to turn your legs to your left side until they're parallel to the ground.

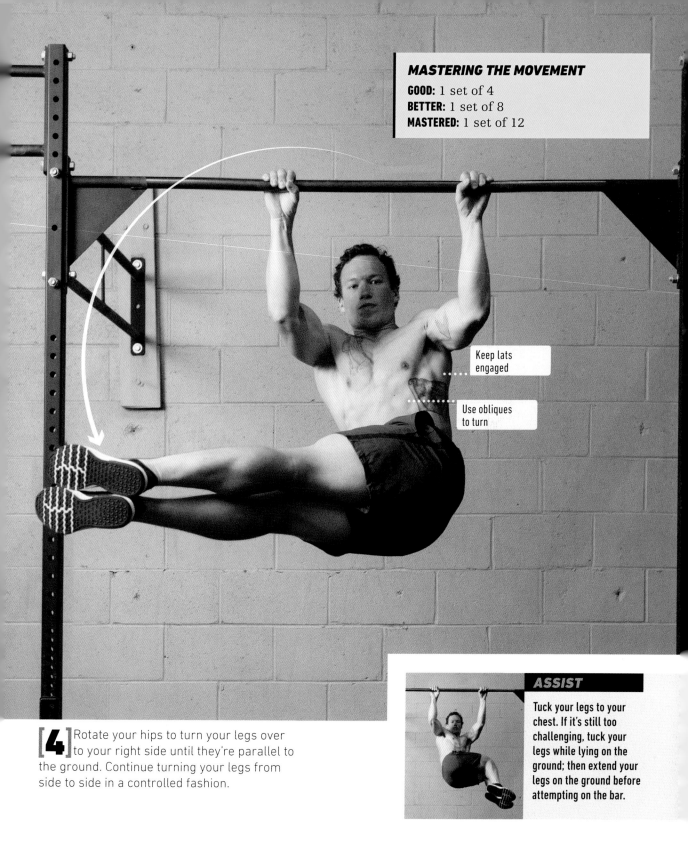

Keep lats
engaged

Use obliques
to turn

ASSIST

Tuck your legs to your chest. If it's still too challenging, tuck your legs while lying on the ground; then extend your legs on the ground before attempting on the bar.

[4] Rotate your hips to turn your legs over to your right side until they're parallel to the ground. Continue turning your legs from side to side in a controlled fashion.

FLYING CROW

The Flying Crow is a traditional yoga pose, but it's also an absolute killer for increasing upper-body strength, improving hip flexibility and mobility, and generating critical balance skills.

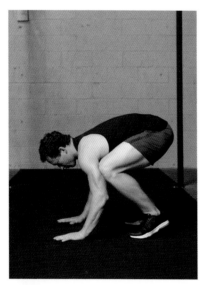

[1] Begin in a squatting position with your hands placed flat on the ground in front of you and positioned shoulder width apart. Position your feet shoulder width apart with your toes aligned directly below your core. Slowly rise up onto your toes until your knees are placed directly against the back of your upper arms. (Your weight should be evenly distributed through your hands and toes.)

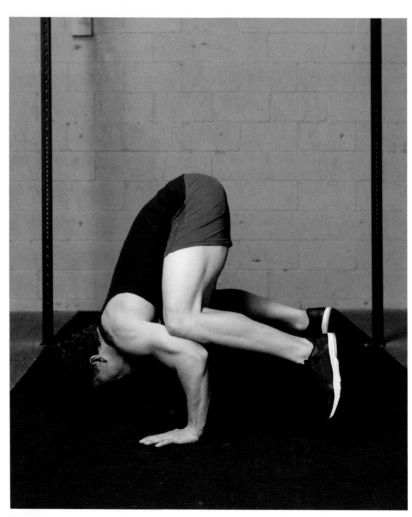

[2] Engage your abdominals to pull your belly up and in toward your back; then roll slightly forward and onto your hands, rounding your spine into a *C* shape until your toes are off the ground and you've completely shifted your weight to your hands.

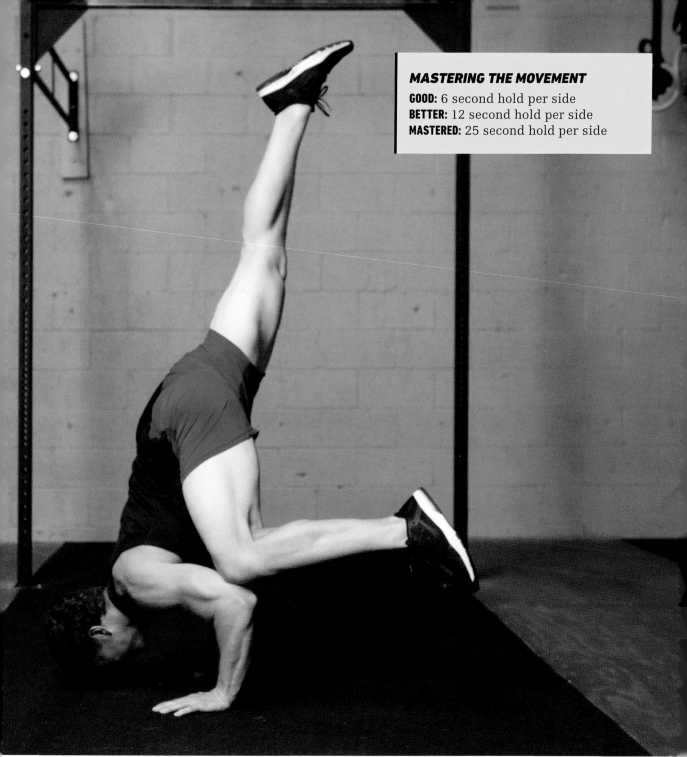

[3] Slowly extend one leg skyward, maintaining your balance. Hold.

SKIN THE CAT

Skin the Cat builds shoulder strength and helps develop a full range of shoulder motion, from full flexion to full extension. This movement can also be done on a chin-up bar.

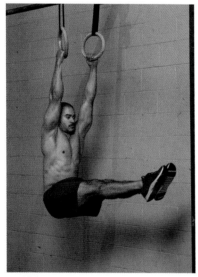

[1] Begin in a dead-hang L-sit position by grasping gymnastic rings with your hands facing in, your arms locked, and your legs fully extended in front of you with your toes pointing forward.

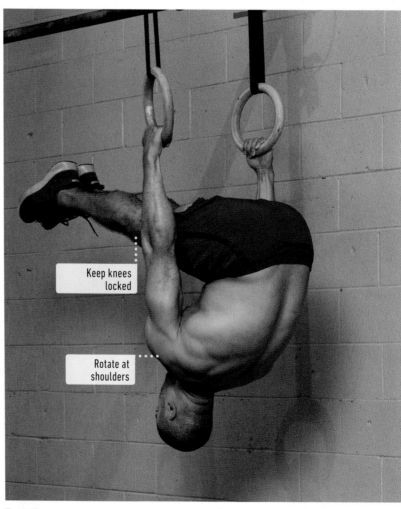

Keep knees locked

Rotate at shoulders

[2] In a controlled fashion, engage your core, pull down on the rings, and pull your hips and legs up over your head and past your arms.

TIP

Begin with the rings positioned low so you can touch your feet to the ground.

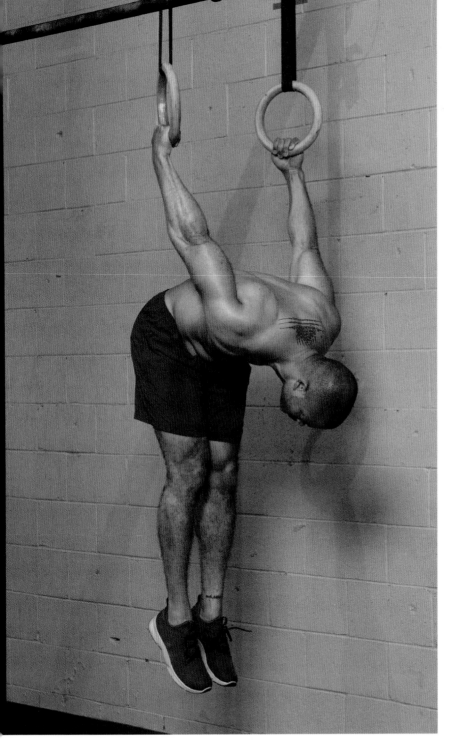

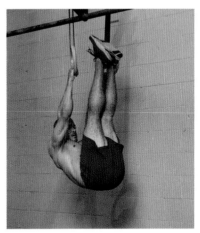

[4] Engage your core and arms, and lift your hips to begin rotating your legs back overhead and in the opposite direction.

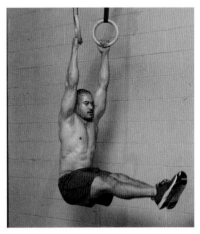

[3] Continue rotating in a controlled fashion until you arrive in a full German hang position.

[5] Continue rotating your legs around until you're back in the starting position.

PLANCHE

The Planche is a truly impressive move that requires superior arm, shoulder, and core strength. Don't rush your training for this one, it will require patience to master.

[1] Begin in a kneeling position in front of a set of parallettes positioned shoulder width apart on the ground. Place your hands in the middle of the grips, and lean forward until your shoulders are in front of your hands.

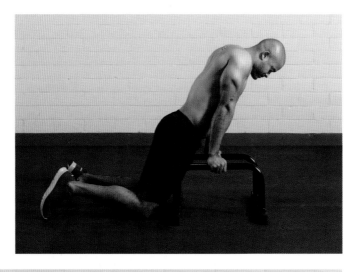

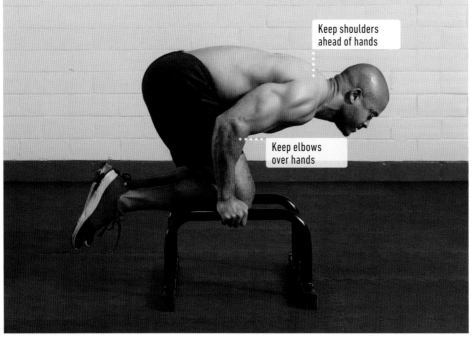

Keep shoulders ahead of hands

Keep elbows over hands

[2] Continue leaning forward and pulling your knees up until your toes leave the ground and your knees are positioned below your chest in a tuck planche position.

Keep back straight

Lock knees

Lock elbows

[3] Slowly extend your arms to push your body up, and then extend one leg at a time until both legs are in a full straddle position. Hold.

INDEX

#

180 Rocket Jump, 122–123

A

Ab Crunch Shredder, 100–101
Air Squat, 150–151
All-4-1 workout, 31
Archer Pull-Up, 80–81

B

band stretching, 20
body positioning, 18
Bodyweight Row, 66–67
Box Jump, 134–135
Box-to-Broad Jump, 140–141
breakfast, 17
Brick by Brick workout, 27
Broad Jump, 138–139
Build the Foundation workout, 26
Bullet-Proof Core workout, 28
Burpee, 128–129
Buzzsaw, 102–103

C

calisthenics, 10
    benefits, 12–13
cardio movements
    180 Rocket Jump, 122–123
    Box Jump, 134–135
    Box-to-Broad Jump, 140–141
    Broad Jump, 138–139
    Burpee, 128–129
    Carioca Run, 124–125
    Half Burpee, 118–119
    Hurricane Burpee, 130–131
    Jumping Lunge, 126–127
    Lateral Hurdle Jump, 136–137
    Skater, 120–121
    Sumo Squat Jump, 132–133
Carioca Run, 124–125
Chin-Up, 68–69
Clapping Pull-Up, 82–83
Clapping Push-Up, 46–47
Commando Pull-Up, 74–75
core movements
    Ab Crunch Shredder, 100–101
    Buzzsaw, 102–103
    Dragon Flag, 106–107
    Front Lever, 110–111
    Hanging Knee Raise, 92–93
    Hanging Leg Raise, 96–97
    Headstand Leg Raise, 104–105
    Human Flag, 114–115
    L-Sit, 98–99
    Oblique Starfish, 94–95
    Tuck Human Flag, 112–113
    Tuck Lever, 108–109
Cræft workout, 30
Crucifix Push-Up, 60–61

D

Dip to L-Sit, 56–57
Double-Leg Mountain Climber, 174–175
Dragon Walk, 178–179
dynamic warm-up, 18

E

Elevated Single-Leg Glute Bridge, 156–157
"empty mind" technique, 15
equipment, 13, 22
    foam rollers, 22
    kettlebells, 22
    mobility ball, 22
    parallettes, 23
    plyo box, 23
    power bands, 23
exercises
    180 Rocket Jump, 122–123
    Ab Crunch Shredder, 100–101
    Air Squat, 150–151
    Archer Pull-Up, 80–81
    Bodyweight Row, 66–67
    Box Jump, 134–135
    Box-to-Broad Jump, 140–141
    Broad Jump, 138–139
    Burpee, 128–129
    Buzzsaw, 102–103
    Carioca Run, 124–125
    Chin-Up, 68–69
    Clapping Pull-Up, 82–83
    Clapping Push-Up, 46–47
    Commando Pull-Up, 74–75
    Crucifix Push-Up, 60–61
    Dip to L-Sit, 56–57
    Double-Leg Mountain Climber, 174–175
    Dragon Flag, 106–107
    Dragon Walk, 178–179
    Elevated Single-Leg Glute Bridge, 156–157
    Explosive Knee Jump, 158–159
    Flying Crow, 182–183
    Front Lever, 110–111
    Glute Bridge and March, 152–153
    Half Burpee, 118–119
    Hamstring Curl, 160–161
    Handstand Push-Up, 62–63
    Hanging Knee Raise, 92–93
    Hanging Leg Raise, 96–97
    Headstand Leg Raise, 104–105
    Human Flag, 114–115
    Hurricane Burpee, 130–131
    Jumping Lunge, 126–127
    Lateral Hurdle Jump, 136–137
    L-Sit, 98–99
    L-Sit Rope Climb, 86–87
    Lunge, 146–147
    Muscle-Up, 84–85
    Ninja Push-Up, 176–177
    Nordic Hamstring Curl, 162–163
    Oblique Starfish, 94–95
    One Arm, One Leg Push-Up, 54–55

One-Arm Pull-Up, 88–89
One-Arm Push-Up, 50–51
One-Hand Clapping Push-Up, 52–53
In-And-Out Grip Pull-Up, 76–77
Pike Push-Up, 44–45
Pistol Squat, 166–167
Planche, 186–187
Pull-Up, 70–71
Push-Up, 38–39
Push-Up with Alternating Leg and Arm Raise, 40–41
Russian Push-Up, 42–43
Shrimp Squat, 164–165
Side Lunge, 148–149
Skater, 120–121
Skin the Cat, 184–185
Sumo Squat Jump, 132–133
Superman Push-Up, 48–49
Triple-Clap Push-Up, 58–59
Tuck Human Flag, 112–113
Tuck Lever, 108–109
Turkish Get-Up, 170–173
Uneven-Grip Pull-Up, 78–79
Wall Sit, 154–155
Weighted Pull-Up, 72–73
Windshield Wiper, 180–181
Explosive Knee Jump, 158–159

F

Flying Crow, 182–183
foam rollers, 22
foam rolling, 20
food as fuel, 16
Front Lever, 110–111
functional training, 11

G

Glute Bridge and March, 152–153
Grind Mode Training Scale, 19

H

Half Burpee, 118–119
Hamstring Curl, 160–161
Handstand Push-Up, 62–63
Hanging Knee Raise, 92–93
Hanging Leg Raise, 96–97
Headstand Leg Raise, 104–105
HGH (Human Growth Hormone), 21
Human Flag, 114–115
Hurricane Burpee, 130–131
hydration, 16

I

In-And-Out Grip Pull-Up, 76–77
injury prevention, 21
Invictus workout, 29

J

Jumping Lunge, 126–127

K

Kaizen, 14–15
kallos, 10
kettlebells, 22

L

Lateral Hurdle Jump, 136–137
leg movements
  Air Squat, 150–151
  Elevated Single-Leg Glute Bridge, 156–157
  Explosive Knee Jump, 158–159
  Glute Bridge and March, 152–153
  Hamstring Curl, 160–161
  Lunge, 146–147
  Nordic Hamstring Curl, 162–163
  Pistol Squat, 166–167
  Shrimp Squat, 164–165
  Side Lunge, 148–149
  Wall Sit, 154–155
L-Sit, 98–99
L-Sit Rope Climb, 86–87
Lunge, 146–147

M

metabolism, managing, 17
mobility ball, 22
muri, 14–15
Muscle-Up, 84–85

N

Nerves of Steel workout, 35
Ninja Push-Up, 176–177
Nordic Hamstring Curl, 162–163
nutrition, 16–17

O

Oblique Starfish, 94–95
One Arm, One Leg Push-Up, 54–55
One-Arm Pull-Up, 88–89
One-Arm Push-Up, 50–51
One-Hand Clapping Push-Up, 52–53

P

pacing workouts, 19, 21
parallettes, 23
Pike Push-Up, 44–45
Pistol Squat, 166–167
Planche, 186–187
plyo box, 23
Popcorn-Ready workout, 34
power bands, 23
progression, training, 18
proprioception, 13
pulling movements
  Archer Pull-Up, 80–81
  Bodyweight Row, 66–67
  Chin-Up, 68–69
  Clapping Pull-Up, 82–83
  Commando Pull-Up, 74–75
  L-Sit Rope Climb, 86–87
  Muscle-Up, 84–85
  One-Arm Pull-Up, 88–89
  In-And-Out Grip Pull-Up, 76–77
  Pull-Up, 70–71
  Uneven-Grip Pull-Up, 78–79
  Weighted Pull-Up, 72–73
Pull-Up, 70–71
pushing movements
  Clapping Push-Up, 46–47
  Crucifix Push-Up, 60–61
  Dip to L-Sit, 56–57
  Handstand Push-Up, 62–63
  One-Arm, One-Leg Push-Up, 54–55
  One-Arm Push-Up, 50–51
  One-Hand Clapping Push-Up, 52–53
  Pike Push-Up, 44–45
  Push-Up, 38–39
  Push-Up with Alternating Leg and Arm Raise, 40–41

Russian Push-Up, 42–43
Superman Push-Up,
48–49
Triple-Clap Push-Up,
58–59
Push-Up, 38–39
Push-Up with
Alternating Leg and
Arm Raise, 40–41
pyramid, training, 18

R

recovery techniques, 20
Redistribution workout,
32
Russian Push-Up, 42–43

S

Shrimp Squat, 164–165
Side Lunge, 148–149
Skater, 120–121
Skin the Cat, 184–185
sleep, proper hygiene,
21
starvation, 16
sthénos, 10
Sumo Squat Jump,
132–133
Superman Push-Up,
48–49

T

trigger pointing, 20
Triple-Clap Push-Up,
58–59
True Grit workout, 33
Tuck Human Flag,
112–113
Tuck Lever, 108–109
Turkish Get-Up, 170–173

U

Uneven-Grip Pull-Up,
78–79

V

Varying workouts, 19

W

Wall Sit, 154–155
warm-up, dynamic, 18
weigh-ins, 17
Weighted Pull-Up, 72–73
whole foods, 17
whole-body movements
Double-Leg Mountain
Climber, 174–175
Dragon Walk, 178–179
Flying Crow, 182–183
Ninja Push-Up, 176–177
Planche, 186–187
Skin the Cat, 184–185
Turkish Get-Up, 170–173
Windshield Wiper,
180–181
whole-body workouts
All-4-1, 31
Brick by Brick, 27
Build the Foundation, 26
Bullet-Proof Core, 28
Cræft, 30
Invictus, 29
Nerves of Steel, 35
Popcorn-Ready, 34
Redistribution, 32
True Grit, 33
Windshield Wiper,
180–181

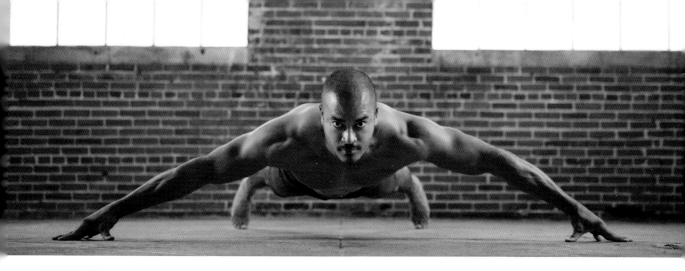

ABOUT THE AUTHOR

TEE MAJOR is a fitness coach and elite-level athlete whose philosophy is centered around building power and strength with only minimal equipment and no machines. Tee is an ACE-certified Group Fitness Trainer with specializations in fitness, nutrition, and tactical strength and conditioning. Tee has trained active-duty service personnel from all major branches of the United States military, as well as professional athletes, Olympians, and everyday people from all walks of life. Find Tee online at www.teemajor.com.

AUTHOR'S ACKNOWLEDGMENTS

Creating this book has been one of the most rewarding and humbling experiences of my life. Every day I hope I make those who love me and look up to me proud.

This writing journey was a true test of creativity and focus. I would have never been able to pull it off without the guidance, patience, and organization of Brook Farling, and the team at Alpha and DK. Big shout out to Kyle Curran, Megan Ridley, and Hudson Wikoff for adding some much-needed abs and beauty to the book. I'm so happy you were a part of this.

To U.S. military special operators Colonel Jerime L. Reid and Colonel Shirlene DelaCruz Santiago Ostrov for the use of your troops, for honoring me with the duty of guiding them to become their best, and for allowing me the space to become my best self in the process.

To my mother, nothing I have done up until this point in my life would have been possible without your love and strength. Your love got me here, and your strength keeps me going. Special thanks to my father, Thomas Major, for instilling discipline and having the foresight to purchase the IBM PS/1 for our home when I was just 8 years old.

Thank you to Jillian Michaels for being kind, caring, and inspirational, and to JLH and family for planting seeds of hope, wisdom, and love.

I would have never been able to accomplish any of this without my loving wife Lilia's kindness, and her reminder that I must be kind to my body, as well. Without you I would be a broken man. Every love story is beautiful, but ours is my favorite.

PUBLISHER'S ACKNOWLEDGMENTS

DK and Alpha Books would like to thank Megan Ridley, Hudson Wikoff, and Kyle Curran for lending their modeling talents to the book. DK and Alpha Books would also like to thank Peter Brasovan and Jared Byczko of Naptown Fitness for allowing us the use of their facility, and Todd Mattingly of Brandt Construction for allowing us the use of their facility.

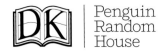

Publisher Mike Sanders
Associate publisher Billy Fields
Senior editor Brook Farling
Book designer William Thomas
Photographer Elese Bales
Art director Nigel Wright
Prepress technician Ayanna Lacey
Proofreader Monica Stone
Indexer Brad Herriman

First American Edition, 2018
Published in the United States by DK Publishing
345 Hudson Street, New York, New York 10014

A catalog record for this book
is available from the Library of Congress.
ISBN 978-1-4654-7351-6

DK books are available at special discounts when purchased
in bulk for sales promotions, premiums, fund-raising, or educational
use. For details, contact: DK Publishing Special Markets, 345 Hudson
Street, New York, New York 10014
SpecialSales@dk.com

Printed and bound in China

A WORLD OF IDEAS:
SEE ALL THERE IS TO KNOW

www.dk.com